"In *Beyond Normal*, Shai Efrati shares gripping accounts of the meticulous medical science that has driven his series of unlikely discoveries with hyperbaric oxygen therapy over the past nearly twenty years. Shai and his brilliant team have shown how the body's natural biochemistry can, through a molecular response known as the hyperoxic-hypoxic paradox, stimulate a surge of stem cells, mitochondria, and new blood flows that repair patients once severely weakened by stroke, concussion, fibromyalgia, PTSD, and Long COVID. Many of their stories are here. If you or anyone you know suffers from any of these diseases, this book will be a lifeline. *Beyond Normal* stands as a milestone, a turning point in the science and clinical medicine of healthy aging and brain research."

> —NIR BARZILAI, MD, founding director, Institute for Aging Research at the Albert Einstein College of Medicine, and author of *Age Later: Health Span, Life Span, and the New Science of Longevity*

"Even though Thomas Kuhn's *The Structures of Scientific Revolutions* suggests paradigm shifts (whether Copernican, Newtonian, chemical, or Einsteinian, to name a few) don't occur very often, *Beyond Normal* certainly appears to be one in neuroscience. In fact, calling Shai Efrati's book and what it represents a game-changer in neuroscience is a huge understatement. The scientific evidence presented here and the proof that hyperbaric oxygen therapy transforms lives and enhances performance is indisputable. It clearly represents a tipping point that takes neuroplasticity to a whole new level and gives everyone hope!"

> —WILLIAM J. CARL, PHD, international lecturer on the brain at medical schools and medical conferences, former president of Pittsburgh Theological Seminary, and author of espionage thriller *Assassin's Manuscript*

BEYOND NORMAL

amplify
an imprint of Amplify Publishing Group

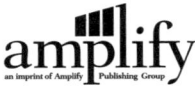

www.amplifypublishinggroup.com

Beyond Normal: How the New Science of Enhanced Medicine Elevates Peak Performance and Repairs Brain Injuries

Image Credits:
Page 25: Aviv Clinics
Page 28: NASCAR Euro
Page 32: Aviv Clinics
Page 35: Joseph C. Maroon, MD
Page 39: Wix.com.
Page 50: Allstar Picture Library Ltd / Alamy Stock Photo (above left); Abaca Press / Alamy Stock Photo (top); PA Images / Alamy Stock Photo (above right)
Page 71: Aviv Clinics
Page 80: Mark N. Miller-UCSF, PhD, Brainard Lab (LEFT); Credit to Virgo Consortium for Cosmological Supercomputer Simulations (RIGHT)
Page 175: Aviv Clinics
All other images: Sagol Center for Hyperbaric Medicine and Research, Israel

For more information, please contact:
Amplify Publishing, an imprint of Amplify Publishing Group
620 Herndon Parkway, Suite 220
Herndon, VA 20170
info@amplifypublishing.com

Library of Congress Control Number: 2024906397

CPSIA Code: PRV0624A

ISBN-13: 979-8-89138-150-6

Printed in the United States

BEYOND NORMAL

HOW THE NEW SCIENCE OF ENHANCED MEDICINE ELEVATES PEAK PERFORMANCE AND REPAIRS BRAIN INJURIES

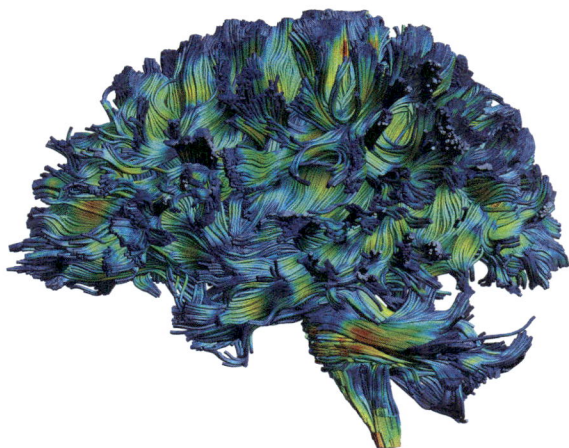

SHAI EFRATI, MD

with Thomas C. Hayes

amplify

an imprint of Amplify Publishing Group

CONTENTS

PART I

BEYOND NORMAL

CHAPTER 1

The Dawning of Enhanced Medicine

I will never forget the first time I saw a middle-aged woman who had been in a wheelchair for five years stand up and walk out of the hospital under her own power.

That's not supposed to happen, I thought.

It was 2005, and she was in the hospital regularly for treatments in a hyperbaric oxygen chamber to heal diabetic ulcers on her legs, but that regimen was unrelated to the stroke years before that had left her unable to use them.

Those improved oxygen supplies were effective. *That* was expected. But a disabled stroke patient suddenly walking? No.

Shai, there are things you don't understand, I reminded myself. *Just continue with your life.*

At the time, I was a resident in nephrology at Assaf Harofeh (now Shamir) Medical Center, one of the top hospitals in Israel. My plan was to dedicate my career to research and treatment of patients with kidney problems. I knew about hyperbaric oxygen therapy because I was a recreational diver but didn't regard it as a specialty worth pursuing.

But then the same scene unfolded a second time, and then a third time: a patient who had received repeated hyperbaric oxygen treatments for diabetic wounds had recovered some physical movement or speaking capacity that had been previously lost due to a stroke.

I took a few deep breaths and shook my head. *Oh shit*, I thought. *This doesn't make sense to me, but . . . it doesn't necessarily need to make sense to me. The knowledge and data I have so far may be limited, not permitting me to see something as it really is.*

Was it possible that the biochemical repair mechanism healing wounds in the legs has a similar impact in the brain? Can this mechanism repair what medical science considered *chronic* brain damage from stroke? It seemed so to me. But nothing meaningful in the medical literature I found had seriously explored this.

I had to solve this puzzle.

It was never my intention to investigate or treat disorders such as stroke, concussion, fibromyalgia, post-traumatic stress disorder (PTSD), Long COVID, or possibly even Alzheimer's disease. (We examine each of these in separate chapters in Part II). But I have been doing it now for nearly twenty years as director of the Sagol Center for Hyperbaric Medicine and Research.

What we've discovered in our research—which is centered on hyperbaric treatment but goes far beyond—has the potential to be revolutionary.

The Problem with "Normal"

In modern medicine, physicians usually default to "normal" as a desired outcome when treating patients. In other words, in traditional medicine, "normal" is considered an average condition for a patient based on their age and sex.

I will never forget the overwhelming joy of two parents on the day their daughter was able to move a finger for the first time in years and to blink her eyes in response to simple yes-or-no questions.

In her early thirties, she had suffered a severe brain injury, unable to communicate in any way following a tragic accident years before. Her parents had struggled with devastating grief ever since.

I was thrilled that night while driving to my home outside Tel Aviv. If a medical intervention can produce a change so basic as pointing a finger and blinking an eye—and unleash this powerful emotional response I had just witnessed—why should physicians be the ones to determine what a good result from treatment should be? This woman's primitive communication mode was far below "normal for her age," yet her parents celebrated.

I will also never forget watching on television one of the many athletes we support at our clinics, the outstanding Israeli judoka Peter Paltchik, joyfully raising Olympic bronze medals and Israel's white-and-blue Star of David flag with his teammates in the mixed-team competition.

That achievement touched off a wave of national pride that lasted for days. Judo became the national sport of Israel. And that made me think, *Isn't it time for physicians and medical scientists who study biology to dedicate more of their energy and resources toward enhancing human performance? To apply our rapidly developing insights in molecular biology, the workings of our bodies' tiniest building blocks, the cells?* We can help people act on their ambition to enjoy better health and better lives . . . far beyond the "normal" for their age.

And I will never forget my first clinical patient with PTSD. Like millions of people diagnosed with PTSD, he had thought that the blame was on him for his feelings of confusion and despair, that he had not been doing all he should be doing to cure himself, and that his "mental disability" had nothing to do with his biology. Until we showed him otherwise.

Sitting before me, he said, as if he were dreaming, "I used to have PTSD, but . . . now I don't have it anymore."

By then our research had led us to understand that mental illness may be rooted in tissue damaged in the brain regions responsible for what we call "mental/psychological behavior." And that psychological trauma alone, with no corresponding tangible injury, might trigger damage to brain cells just like any physical injury suffered from a car accident, gunshot, or explosion. I wondered, *What is the biology underlying what we too often interpret as mental disorder?*

Each of these four intense personal experiences begged two important questions: Why should physicians default to "normal" as a desired outcome when treating patients? Why not aim for the best any patient's current physiological and biological condition can allow?

My obsession with these questions spurred me to develop a new way for doctors and society to think about how we administer healthcare. I call it *enhanced medicine.* Enhanced medicine is about not only treating injuries but making our bodies and minds reach the best of their biological potential.

Our starting point with clients or patients as physicians practicing enhanced medicine is this: "Tell us your biological wish, and we will see if we can make it happen."

We want to help you reach higher levels of performance regardless of what you are able to do now. From wheelchair-bound paraplegics to the world's greatest athletes, the goals of enhanced medicine are to help you improve from wherever you are now.

Some patients who approach us are in the prime of their lives, with no significant measurable or detectable health issues. They simply want to discover their peak performance; they want to push their boundaries. In these cases, we aren't working to solve issues so much as we're looking to mine untapped potential in their bodies and minds.

Other patients come to us for healing—physical, mental, and emotional. They struggle with issues such as stroke, concussion syndrome, fibromyalgia, PTSD, Long COVID, and even early stages of Alzheimer's disease, which are all issues we'll look at more deeply in Part II. Many are looking to improve worsening and debilitating symptoms from these diseases. They want more autonomy in their lives to complete basic tasks, like dressing themselves or staying active.

It doesn't matter if you are twenty, forty, sixty, eighty years old, or beyond. We want to apply advancing disciplines of medical science and the arts of medicine to enhance your physiological and biological capacity to the maximal potential.

The Four Principles of Enhanced Medicine

FIRST PRINCIPLE: *We want to enhance your physiology and biology to the highest levels you can achieve from whatever those levels are at the outset.*

If you already perform at a high level, such as company chief executives or world-class athletes, the goal of enhanced medicine is to elevate further your physical and mental capacities, to help you think even more clearly or compete with even more power, stamina, and energy.

At the other extreme, if your physical or mental capabilities are way below average—maybe you suffered a stroke or massive brain injury—enhanced medicine should be favorable even if the impact leaves you still below average.

SECOND PRINCIPLE: *Our interventions focus intensely on finding and removing bottlenecks that prevent your biology, at the cellular level, from performing.*

What do I mean by bottlenecks? Bottlenecks are biological obstacles to better performance. For example, when blood vessels become blocked or substantially narrowed from accumulated cholesterol, the restricted supply of blood and oxygen weakens the performance of all cells downstream from that blockage. Then, too, cell performance falls if the power generators of cells, the mitochondria, malfunction in some way. Removing these and myriad other bottlenecks triggers a cascade of restorative physiological and biological responses.

In classical medicine, which is what most medical schools teach, physicians are trained to target a single troublesome enzyme or receptor using a specific drug. For example, an antibiotic is used to treat a specific bacterium. In enhanced medicine, we do use drugs embraced by classical medicine, but we have a broader intent—to trigger our whole body to function in a better way. Vaccination is a wonderful example of this.

Vaccination is a type of enhanced medicine. In effect, we inject a weakened bacteria into the body so the immune system can recognize this new invader and attack the more dangerous version after an infection. The approach in classical medicine is to use an antibiotic to treat a disease caused by an infection from those same bacteria, but *after* the infection. The vaccine keeps you safe from contracting that disease in the first place.

THIRD PRINCIPLE: *Everything we do should be measured: quantified before and after the intervention.*

Why is this important? We need to make sure that whatever improvement we are targeting in someone's health, in their biology, is achieved. We know that different interventions can induce different biological effects on different individuals. What may be true for the general population may not hold for the specific client we are treating. In the vaccination example, for instance, we expect the immune system to be better prepared after a vaccination to ward off disease from that bacterial infection.

Blood tests enable us to measure and monitor the presence of antibodies and certain immune cells designed by the immune system to seek and destroy those bacteria. Or, if our goal is to achieve better brain functionality through hyperbaric oxygen therapy (an important part of the enhanced medicine tool kit we'll explore shortly), we can monitor that before and after the intervention by high-resolution functional imaging of the brain and by computerized cognitive tests.

FOURTH PRINCIPLE: *Enhanced medicine starts with effective communication with clients.*

We need to invest the time necessary to understand the whole picture, including the client's personal life. Our first priority is listening to understand clearly what the client needs. The second priority flows from that understanding: sketching, in detail, a realistic, achievable biological outcome for the client.

One of the most important skills for any physician is conducting a medical interview. This requires booking enough time for that discussion, often a half hour or more. In the United States and many other countries, committing a half hour or more for patient interviews is a real challenge. Most physicians have so many patients that they cannot spend more than ten or fifteen minutes with each one. They do not have time to explore any condition in detail. Prescribing a pill requires the least amount of time with a patient. So, what happens? Most often, physicians prescribe a pill.

In contrast, evaluations and interventions in enhanced medicine are time-consuming. This time commitment is crucial for physicians and clients to achieve their specific goals. Physicians practicing enhanced medicine need to invest time with people in their care to gather insights and updates about their experience. Physicians should be prepared to put everything on the table when they meet a patient and to encourage an open discussion.

Let's say, for example, that you have had a stroke and now are considering a program in enhanced medicine. Our first steps before treatment would be analyzing state-of-the-art functional and structural images of your brain, then compiling a comprehensive physical and cognitive evaluation of your brain. At that point, we would explain in simple, nontechnical terms to you what we believe we can achieve.

As you might expect, it takes time to walk through and translate, in simple terms, all the analyses and evaluations we assembled and the questions and prospects for treatment that they raise. We might see, for example, a high probability to improve your ability to think but not your motor skills. Would you be willing to accept that outcome? Would you want to proceed with an enhanced medicine program, or not?

Our purpose—our imperative, really—in taking these initial steps is to establish high levels of trust that are necessary to customize the deep knowledge and medical technologies available now for treating patients or clients in enhanced medicine.

The Six Core Disciplines of Enhanced Medicine

1. Hormesis

- Hormesis plays a crucial role in enhanced medicine, generating a signal to help prepare the body for the next stressor events. It is a grand idea and a grand bargain: to induce stress in the body for a positive biological change. We are fine-tuning the body, preparing for physical challenges you expect.

• The basic concept is to expose your body to a specific stress in low "doses"—in a safe, controlled way that is below some higher level that could cause real damage. This requires a controlled exposure to a stress. You need to stress your body for it to work better, to enhance your performance. That is what I mean by a "grand bargain." The goal is to trigger your biology to function better to reach your biological goal.

• We condition our whole body at the cellular level to be ready for an array of biological challenges that may arise. You cannot just go out some day with no prior training and run a 10k as fast as you can and expect to avoid injury. You prepare for the run over time by, in effect, triggering your biology to adjust with a controlled lower "dose" of rising stressors in distance, tempo, and speed. Otherwise, you will risk stress fractures, torn muscles, and other injuries, and you will not reach your biological goals to help you run a faster, injury-free race.

• The grand bargain is to push yourself, to induce stress in limited amounts similar to what you anticipate during the race. You don't run at maximum speed longer than these limited bursts because you don't want to accelerate the stress to a point where you risk injury.

• Fast runs up to a distance of 100 yards that approach your maximum speed—sprints known as striders—are an example of controlled exposure. The physical exertion during these sprints prepares all the cells in your body—heart, lungs, liver, kidneys, stomach, and more—to achieve the pace goal you set for upcoming races. It is more than a matter of conditioning the bone, muscle, and ligaments in your lower body.

- Consider again our vaccination example. Being vaccinated with a small dose of weakened bacteria or virus is another way of using hormesis to achieve a certain biological goal. The weak quantities of a virus or bacteria injected into your bloodstream train your immune system in advance to defend against the more potent virus or bacteria, should you encounter it. As we noted before, in classical medicine you are given an antibiotic or other medicine after you are already sick.

Misconceptions, Fallacies, Rejections

Hormesis has a bad reputation among some medical professionals for at least three reasons. First, the basics of hormesis are not taught in medical school. Most practicing physicians are not familiar with the concepts or the science and, as a result, they are often skeptical about its principles and approach.

Then, too, practitioners of homeopathic medicine made unsubstantiated claims that extremely small doses of undetectable toxic biochemicals will train your body to ward off illness. The homeopathic practitioners lauded these undetectable and unmeasured levels of toxic biochemicals as examples of hormesis at work, of how the body can heal itself. They were not.

The final point, which relates closely to the first, is that even among physicians who are aware of hormesis, most do not incorporate the concepts and science of hormesis into their own lives. Many lack the knowledge and motivation required to do this. Thus, they are not able to be genuine advocates for hormesis. If asked, they cannot reply positively to the simple question, "Are you doing it yourself?"

2. Physical Exercise

The physiological, biological, and mental benefits of intermittent physical exercise, of course, have been extensively investigated by scientists, physiologists, and other professionals. Millions of people have embraced these findings to improve their health and well-being. The benefits are legion.

- Let's look at two key points about intermittent physical exercise that explain its crucial role in enhanced medicine programs: One is hormesis, preparing the body at the cellular level to meet the next physical challenge. Physical exercise builds more mitochondria, more muscles, more blood vessels. It improves your heart's capacity to pump more blood through the body, enabling your mitochondria to process more oxygen and generate more energy. These benefits to your physiology and biology happen not during the exercise itself but between exercise sessions. That is why physicians, nurses, physical therapists, and well-trained coaches preach that recovery time is crucial for athletes.

- If you take physical exercise or training to the extreme—without taking recovery days in between—you risk breaking bones, major tissue injuries, endless inflammation, and more. Your physical condition will decline. However, if you exercise for a certain period of time—not continuously, not every day of the week—and then follow with recovery periods, these various exercises build strength and endurance. In hormesis terms, they induce resilience to the next stressor. As we build resilience to stressors through an ongoing, regular exercise schedule, the body prepares itself for this repetitive event.

- The second point is that when you exercise, there are immediate, direct benefits that flow from your body's natural biochemistry. For example, exercise may directly affect areas of the brain, such as the amygdala and prefrontal cortex, that are rich in receptors for endocannabinoids and that regulate the stress response.

- Endocannabinoids have the same chemical compounds found in cannabis, the marijuana plant: the "don't worry, be happy" chemicals. Endocannabinoid molecules reduce anxiety and induce a state of contentment when they lock into these receptors in the amygdala and prefrontal cortex. Endocannabinoids also increase dopamine in the brain's reward system, further fueling sensations of optimism.

- Osteocalcin, a hormone, is another example of how exercise produces biochemical benefits in the brain. During workouts, your bones manufacture and release osteocalcin into your bloodstream. In the brain, osteocalcin helps sharpen your thinking by improving brain function and memory. Osteocalcin has many other known benefits beyond the brain, such as making energy more available in muscles, improving male fertility, and promoting absorption of glucose into liver, fat, and skeletal muscle cells.

3. Nutrition, Diet, and Fasting

The design of different diet regimens should be matched carefully with whatever biological goal we aim to achieve.

- Just as the quality of the fuel we pump into our car affects engine performance and the efficiency of fuel lines, the food that we take into our bodies has a huge effect on the performance of our mitochondria (those cellular engines that convert oxygen to energy), blood vessels ("fuel lines" that carry oxygen to the mitochondria), and hormones (connecting signals that orchestrate the performance of different organs). The amount of food we eat—and the frequency—are factors just as important in shaping the impact of our diets as food quality.

- When not to eat is as important as when to eat. *What?!* you might be thinking. *Even if I'm hungry late at night or early in the morning?* I've learned to anticipate this puzzled response from clients and patients. Many of us learn from an early age that if we're hungry, we should eat something if we can to ease the hunger. We learn that hunger is bad, a signal from the body to our brain. Well, hunger is not bad for limited periods. It is another illustration of hormesis: inducing stress in the body for a positive biological change. Let me explain.

- Intermittent fasting is a discipline that encourages us to eat main meals within a limited time span each day, and then go cold turkey—no snacks, no light meals—at other times. I use an eight-hour time window for eating and fast the other sixteen hours. Intermittent fasting induces a controlled stress as hunger emerges; that is, as the body gradually craves more nutrients, more food. This limited "hunger stress" helps mitochondria to better convert oxygen to energy, and cells to better synthesize new molecules and process other aspects of cell metabolism and resilience. Intermittent fasting also helps the body clean out the garbage accumulated within our cells—a process known as *autophagy*. When we fast roughly twelve hours or more, our cells start consuming unnecessary or dysfunctional components as food. "Auto" means self and "phagy" means eat, so the literal meaning of autophagy is "self-eating."

- Think of it this way: If you eat more of that cream cake in the refrigerator and not the vegetables nearby, over time the vegetables will rot, smell bad, and make all food in the refrigerator unappetizing. However, if all you see in the refrigerator is vegetables, you have no other choice if you are hungry. You will eat them. This is what happens in your cells after twelve hours of fasting.

- We will get into details of my personal regimen for hyperbaric oxygen therapy sessions, fitness, nutrition, and diet in chapter 13.

4. Immune System

- Our immune system plays a crucial role in many chronic illnesses in addition to diseases caused by a specific invading pathogen (bacteria, virus, or fungal). Diseases such as lupus, multiple sclerosis, or rheumatoid arthritis, for example, are triggered by an overzealous immune system that attacks healthy cells, tissues, and other normal parts of the body. On the other hand, when the immune system is generally weak, our body is more vulnerable to invasion and damage from external pathogens. Moreover, our body's capacity to regenerate or repair tissues harmed by any illness or injury is also severely damaged.

- We have also learned in recent years more about the immune system's significant role in fighting cancer cells and the rise of immunotherapy treatments to attack tumor cells. The immune system's resilience or weakness also is a factor in many age-related declines of our physiological and biological functions.

- Immune system resilience—and how we should preserve and enhance it for specific biological goals—will be examined closely as we move through different chapters of the book.

5. Hyperbaric Oxygen Therapy (HBOT)

Hyperbaric oxygen therapy treatments, known as HBOT, are one of the most powerful elements we have in enhanced medicine. HBOT has two primary benefits as well. One is to overcome one of the more common bottlenecks our bodies develop over time: atherosclerosis, a reduced capacity of our cardiovascular system to deliver oxygen to our cells due to the narrowing passageways in our vessels as plaque deposits accumulate and constrict blood flow.

The second is another form of hormesis. One of the most powerful biochemical triggers for the regenerative-repair cascade we prize in enhanced medicine is hypoxia, the lack of oxygen. For that reason, we mimic hypoxia in our hyperbaric oxygen chambers by generating a fast decline from a very high level of oxygen back to the normal level. In these carefully monitored conditions, hypoxia becomes a safe control stressor.

As the body interprets the fast decline from a very high oxygen level to a normal level as hypoxia, it activates a set of responses we call the "hyperoxic–hypoxic paradox" or HHP. This activates multiple biochemical mechanisms to repair whatever new damage the body senses happening from hypoxia, the oxygen deprivation.

Generating HHP through the protocols of HBOT elevates our biochemistry in four remarkable ways. It enables us to (1) dramatically increase the volume of mitochondria; (2) make mitochondria's capacity to convert oxygen to energy more efficient; (3) accelerate the production and migration of stem cells; and (4) generate new blood vessels where blood flows have been reduced.

The HHP component is at the core of why HBOT can be a powerful tool, an important biochemical insight that we'll examine more closely in chapter 3. It shifts the balance from the degeneration of your physical condition (injuries or diseases that take your biology down and the normal decline we experience as we age chronologically) to regeneration (repair and growth).

6. Mental Perception and Resilience

I always teach my students that different people can share the same environment, yet they sense and experience that environment in totally different ways. This is because our perceptions of the world and the more immediate environment we live in are sorted out in our brains. We can go even further: you yourself can experience what appears to be the exact same environment in dramatically different ways at different times in your life.

Picture in your mind several people waiting in line to buy ice cream at Disney World. A child who catches your eye is appealingly curious, enjoying the faces surrounding her and the voices she hears. She delights in the waiting. Yet that same person will react in dramatically different ways to the same stimuli if years later she has developed PTSD after her military service. Now, those nearby faces and voices provoke waves of fear, even terror. Her dread from that moment will affect all her biological functions and, in fact, all her cells.

Or consider a person who is depressed, lacks a sense of purpose, and has no meaningful plans for his future—regardless of chronological age. It could be someone in their twenties, sixties, or eighties. The regenerative biological capacity for this person will be significantly decreased, and any medical insult—any injury or infectious disease—may lead to significant chronic damage. He may not be capable of making much progress in the other core dimensions of enhanced medicine.

Moreover, take the case of two soldiers who went through the same combat situation, the same horrific life-threatening sequence of events. One developed PTSD. He is debilitated, cannot sleep, cannot concentrate, and cannot focus on a mission. He cannot work, cannot write computer code as he did in the past. He continues to relive the horrifying event again and again—likely for the rest of his life if not treated successfully.

The other soldier did not develop PTSD. Why? The baseline of mental resilience was much higher for the second soldier than the baseline for the first soldier. All of us need this baseline resilience to cope successfully with the many repeated stressful events that we encounter in life. With each stress we encounter, we can either continue to build resilience (hormesis) or slip further toward a breakdown.

The different elements of mental perception and resilience will be discussed as well in following chapters, including exciting break-throughs in imaging technologies that enable us to see and measure markers in the brain for baseline mental resilience.

This is the toolbox of principles and disciplines we have within our grasp, new medical insights and technologies with proven potential to elevate your mental and physical abilities to *your* maximum level. We are now at the dawning of enhanced medicine.

Key Takeaways

The Four Principles

1. Enhance your physiology and biology to the highest levels you can achieve from whatever those levels are at the outset.
2. Focus interventions on finding and removing bottle-necks that prevent your biology from performing.
3. Measure everything before and after the intervention. Health metrics defining a desired outcome based on

average results for the client's age are not relevant in enhanced medicine.
4. Effective communication begins by listening to patients' or clients' perspectives to set goals.

CHAPTER 2

Peak Performance

Wanting a life as good or better than those of the people around you is, for most of us, just part of being human.

In Western societies in particular, our cultures celebrate and reward people who strive to achieve their high potential, especially people willing to invest in the hard work to be the best. They set high goals. They push themselves to live the motto of the Olympic Games: *citius, altius, fortius* (faster, higher, stronger).

Even if a person's health data puts them in a category of normal for their age, physicians should not consider "normal" by itself a valid reason not to intervene medically. People can always ask for more. We expect professional athletes or anyone who wants to win an Olympic medal to ask for more.

We should also be alert for opportunities to further enhance brain function and physical performance of relatively healthy people . . . people whose health data are above average for their age and who want to achieve their highest-possible brain performance.

The four professionals profiled in this chapter are among hundreds of elite performers we've counseled and treated in their personal pursuits, whether for peak performance or more vigorous health. The dominating champion of NASCAR's European race car circuit. A neurosurgeon and sports medicine specialist still competing in triathlons in his eighties. A brilliant technology executive and co-founder of a leader in cloud-based website development tools. One of the UK's most famous rugby players who is now coaching in Dubai.

Alon Day: Europe's "Greatest" NASCAR Champion

When Alon Day came to us in 2019, he already was a highly competitive NASCAR driver on the European circuit, a two-time champion. He also had the distinction of being the first Israeli to compete in a major NASCAR event in the United States. But he wanted to do more: "Every day I would wake up and go into that chamber thinking that I want to be the all-time leader in championships. I want another championship."

Alon was not just above average for his age, he was an outlier—in fantastic physical condition and still maintaining a rigorous fitness regimen at age twenty-seven, years after he left the elite fighter pilot training program of the Israel Defense Forces to pursue auto racing. For example, his VO_2 Max* was high at a ratio of 30.8 milliliters per kilogram even before he began HBOT. I was amazed when I saw his initial test results—not as high as a professional cyclist or runner, but higher than I expected for a race car driver.

---

* Maximal oxygen efficiency volume, known as VO_2 Max, is a key measure of fitness in endurance sports, encompassing cardiorespiratory and muscle fitness. Professional and competitive amateur athletes and their trainers keep a close eye on VO_2 Max. It gauges how much oxygen your body can process during periods of maximum physical exertion.

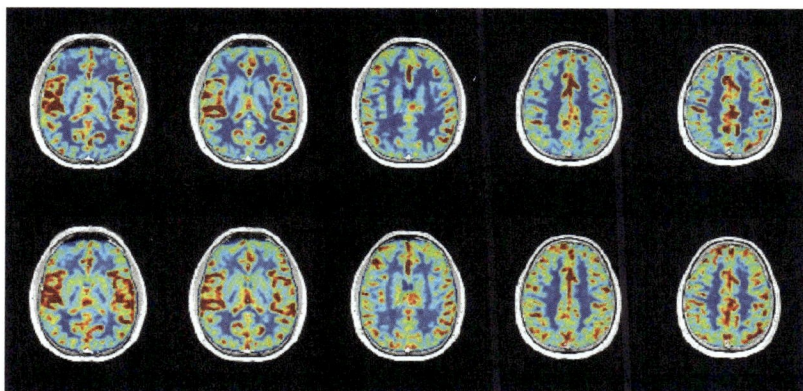

Figure 2-1: Cerebral blood flow (CBF), or perfusion, before Alon's HBOT sessions (upper row) and after (bottom row).

It is true, and probably not widely appreciated, that many NAS-CAR drivers are superior athletes. Racing a car often at speeds reaching nearly 200 miles per hour in hot, cramped confines and wearing a fireproof suit is physically demanding; drivers can lose five pounds or more during a two-hour race. Competitive drivers need superior cardiovascular performance, strength, and stamina to handle the wheel, seize momentary opportunities, avoid sudden calamity (serious injury or even death), execute their strategy, and compete. The pressure is constant and intense.

Yet physical strength and stamina alone are not what sets apart most champions. For elite drivers, physical strength and stamina are table stakes. They can't compete at this level without them. Champions need superior cognitive ability as well. They need lightning-quick mental agility to process new information—a sudden gap opening when a race leader drifts too wide on a turn, or a rival holding pace inches from your right front bumper—and then react instantly and keenly.

"A race car driver needs really good reaction time and high focus," Alon says. "Most professional drivers know neuroscience is an important factor in their performance. When you are racing at 250 to 300 kilometers per hour [approximately 150 to 190 miles per hour], every millisecond counts to whether you finish first or last. The driver's fitness level is really high, but it's not high enough. We get tired during a race, which impairs your focus and your ability to race."

We designed HBOT protocols for Alon to build his cognitive skills in addition to his cardiovascular fitness. As I indicated earlier, young people in their twenties and thirties have abundant stem cell production for physical growth and development. Even so, we can accelerate stem cell production further with the new protocols of hyperbaric oxygen treatment and with selected cognitive drills that are directing rising flows to targeted regions of the brain. We pushed Alon's focus, multitasking, and information-processing speed to the limits. His HBOT training program included memory and reaction training with virtual reality drills.

As he and I discussed at the outset of his treatments, the more rigorously he concentrated on each of the cognitive drills in his program, the more stem cells would be carried to his relevant brain regions, and the more improvement we would see in his brain's processing speed and sharpness. He took advantage, focusing intensely through the treatment program.

His dedication to these drills came naturally. "Since I was ten, I have always been into computer and video games," he says. As a professional race car driver, he often spends two or three hours a day honing his mental agility and other quick-response skills using advanced racing simulators, such as iRacing.

"This trains my brain to adapt more quickly to dynamic situations that happen in racing," he says. "You can change normal factors in a simulator, such as having to make abrupt right turns when the visual is telling you 'Left!' and left turns when the visual says 'Right!' I'll also

Most-Significant CBF Changes					
Brodmann Area	Brain Region	Brain Function	CBF pre -HBOT	CBF post -HBOT	**Percent Change**
7	Superior parietal lobule	Visuo-motor coordination	26.96	38.07	**41.20%**
5	Superior parietal lobule	Somatosensory integration	30.10	42.44	**40.99%**
1	Lateral post-central gyrus	Sensory perception, touch, size, and shape	27.32	37.77	**38.27%**
19	Lateral occipital gyrus	Associative visual cortex	22.32	30.48	**36.55%**
9	Medial frontal gyrus	Working memory, decision-making	30.04	39.99	**33.14%**
46	Dorsolateral prefrontal cortex	Working memory, decision-making	33.77	44.66	**32.24%**
18	Lateral occipital gyrus	Secondary visual cortex	23.40	30.68	**31.12%**
38	Inferior temporal gyrus	Emotion memory	42.16	55.24	**31.03%**

Figure 2-2: Data in the far right column show significant blood flow increases in eight different regions of his brain after Alon's HBOT sessions.

slow the speed of the images to fifteen or twenty frames per second. This forces me to compensate for the missing frames."

The sequence of progressive brain images captured by perfusion MRI-DTI (magnetic resonance imaging and diffusion tensor tractography) during Alon's three months of HBOT (Figure 2-1) shows the benefit of combining HBOT with his singular focus on cognitive drills.

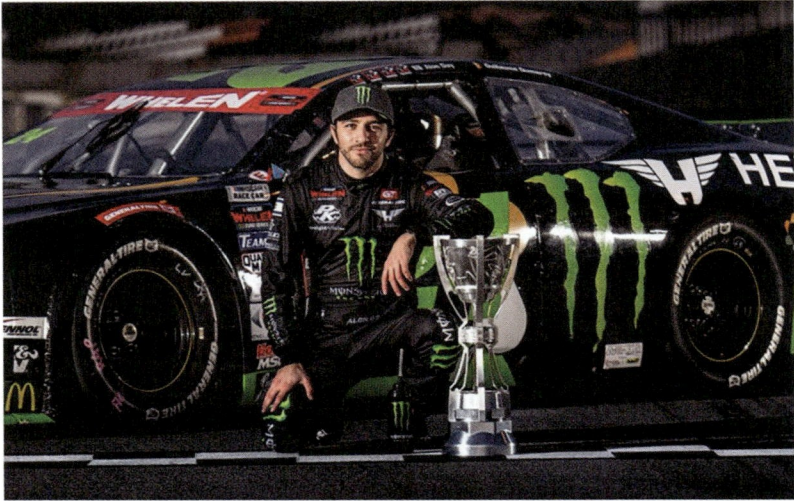

Alon Day with his fourth NASCAR Whelen Euro championship trophy.

"When I saw the changing colors in the MRIs," he says, "it was genuinely exciting."

The more active the brain is, the more perfusion—also known as cerebral blood flow (CBF)—you will have. In the bottom row images in Figure 2-1, you can see more red and more yellow, with red being the higher level of increased perfusion. (The two shades of blue illustrate ventricles filled with fluid they produce and transport in the brain.)

The increased levels of red and yellow (higher perfusion) indicate new blood vessel growth, increased brain metabolism, and changes in the microscopic detail of cells of the relevant brain region.

Alon came to us with an amazing brain. His brain was now functioning at an even *higher* level.

He had worked hard on his virtual reality drills in the chamber. As days passed, "Sitting there breathing oxygen and doing my games, I saw my reaction time in the measurements getting better," he recalls.

"I am the type of person who needs to see proof to back up the feelings. They gave me six sheets of paper detailing the images and measurements of increasing blood flows in my brain. The data after even my first set of three sessions were insane. The measurements showed huge improvements in information processing speed. When I saw the data, I thought: *These are the facts. You can't argue with the facts.*"

At the end of this first HBOT treatment in 2020, Alon won his third NASCAR Whelen Euro Series.

"In motor sports, we always say lap time does the talking. It takes four or five laps for most drivers to get up to full racing speed. Even after the first month of my hyperbaric chamber treatments, I became much faster, getting up to speed quickly, usually within one or two laps. This is where I can really stretch a lead from the pole position or move up if I start back in the field. And I can adapt more quickly to wet tracks or other conditions."

In the 2021 and 2022 racing seasons, he continued extending his NASCAR Whelen record for most cumulative wins to twenty-nine. He had won the champion's trophy an amazing one of every three times in the eighty-seven races he had entered since 2015. The online publication *World of Euro NASCAR* declared Alon had established a "dynasty" in the Euro Series, adding, "Alon Day is perhaps the greatest driver to have competed in NASCAR Whelen Series events."[1]

Weeks before the 2022 summer racing season, Alon began what we describe as "boosting" sessions, his second series of full hyperbaric chamber treatments. "I always search for the extra mile in preparation, somewhere my rivals didn't go," he told us. When the racing season ended that November, Alon had added his *fourth* NASCAR Euro Whelen championship, breaking a tie at three with another driver and raising his cumulative wins to thirty-two.

Rather than compete for a fifth trophy in 2023, Alon took aim at lining up sponsors to back him on a top racing team on NASCAR's premier circuit in the United States. He knows that competition will be unmatched anywhere in the world, but this is what motivates him. "I want to be the best."

Joseph Maroon, MD: Brain Surgeon, Octogenarian Triathlete

Dr. Joseph Maroon is a renowned neurosurgeon and sports medicine specialist perhaps best known for his work with colleagues at the University of Pittsburgh Medical Center (UPMC), treating concussion in thousands of athletes.

More recently, he has investigated with colleagues novel methods in immunotherapy to treat cancer and new approaches to diagnose and treat neurological diseases such as Alzheimer's and Parkinson's. He has served as the team neurosurgeon for the Pittsburgh Steelers for more than four decades, and he remains a Steelers consultant and adviser to the National Football League.

Joe and his late partner in orthopedics, Dr. Freddi Fu, founded the UPMC Sports Medicine Concussion Program in 2003. Its physicians and neuropsychologists evaluate between 7,000 and 8,000 new post-concussion patients each year. Most suffer these injuries in high-impact youth and collegiate sports, such as football, wrestling, basketball, and soccer, but many have been professional race car drivers and football players.

Joe is a remarkable athlete and health and fitness advocate in his own right. He was an Academic All-American football halfback sixty years ago at Indiana University. Later, starting in his late fifties, he completed more than eighty triathlons and eight Ironman distance races (2.4-mile swim, 112-mile bike ride, and 26.2-mile run) before signing up for our three-month treatment program in Florida at eighty-one years old in 2021.

HBOT treatments had consistently helped his post-concussion patients for nearly a decade "when all other modalities had failed," he points out.[2] He was drawn to HBOT initially because he regarded it as an effective treatment for divers suffering the bends, for carbon monoxide poisoning, and for healing peripheral nonhealing diabetic wounds. "When existing treatments fail, I pursue out-of-the-box, innovative treatments. I thought it made sense to use hyperbaric oxygen for brain wounds," he says.[3]

After reading our team's scientific papers on injured and aging brains, he wondered: *Could the full program of enhanced medicine treatments improve my own physical and mental capacities, even as an octogenarian? Could I finish a triathlon faster!?*

"I had read all of their scientific articles prior to making my decision to move to Florida for three months, and I was impressed," he wrote on his blog.[4] "But as a scientist, I still needed objective data proving the benefits were for real. It was a fascinating journey and an experience that I believe has changed my life."

Looking back, he says, the science we developed supporting the efficacy of the HBOT protocol has "facilitated a renaissance in the use of hyperbaric oxygen for brain disorders."[5]

He adds, "I have personally recommended HBOT to numerous patients who have suffered from prolonged post-concussion syndrome with residual headaches, insomnia, vision changes, and foggy thinking. The results have been very positive, with complete resolution of symptoms in many cases."[6]

In that 2022 blog post[7] and a subsequent scientific paper,[8] Joe explains that the HBOT-based treatments elevated his physical energy,

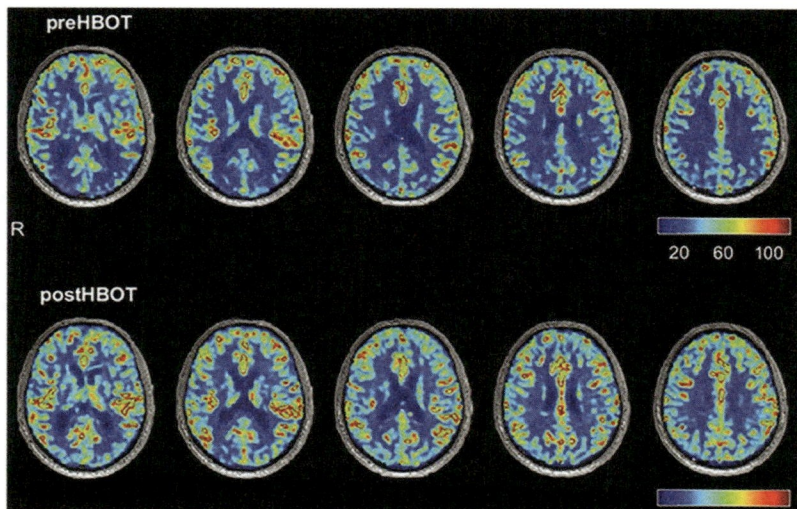

Figure 2-3: These scans show the perfusion pattern in Joe's brain before (top row) and after (bottom row) his HBOT treatments. The increase in yellow and red colors in the bottom row represents increased blood flows.

enabling him to train longer and harder for races, and improved his thought processes and processing speed.

After completing fifty of his sixty HBOT sessions, his triathlon race time was 9 percent faster—*twenty-four minutes faster*—than a previous race he finished before beginning HBOT treatments in Florida.

"I was pretty astounded. My post-race fatigue was less. My muscle soreness was less. My memory was slightly better. My attention to details improved," he recalls.

"I was first in my age group," he told a 2023 conference on hyperbarics medicine, adding wryly, "but I was the only one in my age group!" which was age eighty years and older. In a video interview in

2022, he asserted, "We're going to see more and more athletes utilizing this to supplement their training."[9]

Before committing to the HBOT protocols, he evaluated his own physiological and neurological metrics. He recounted how the treatments improved those metrics in this 2022 peer-reviewed scientific article in *Frontiers in Neurology*: "The effect of hyperbaric oxygen therapy on cognition, performance, proteomics, and telomere length—the difference between zero and one: A case report."

Joe frames the *Frontiers in Neurology* paper about his experience as "a personal case report on a single subject, myself." He adds, "The usefulness of an individual case report like this should not be underestimated because of small sample size when biomarkers provide objective support of the results."

Here, citing data from his treatments, Joe summarizes key physiological gains he experienced.

Physiological Results

- Improvements in anaerobic threshold, exercise endurance, muscle strength, gait speed, and grip strength ranging from 7 to 15 percent

- Improvements in global cognitive function as well as other cognitive function domains in a range of 3.1 to 3.8 percent

- Single-photon emission computerized tomography (SPECT) scans showing increased perfusion in brain areas for memory, ranging from 43.3 to 52.3 percent

- Perfusion MRI showing increases in cerebral perfusion (blood flows) in various functional areas—memory, coordination, and visual motor cortex—ranging from 43.3 to 52.3 percent

- MRI-DTI scans showing increased neuronal connections, ranging from 9 to 22 percent in several white matter areas

What is more, his telomeres length doubled and clusters of inflammatory proteins dropped precipitously at approximately the fortieth session.

This result is highly significant, with promising implications for other normal or above-normal aging individuals. Studies at our Tel Aviv clinic, in addition to HBOT treatment results such as these for Joe and, as we'll see shortly, other clients, have demonstrated that the HBOT protocol lengthens telomeres. When we can halt or reverse the erosion of telomeres, it means that we can target and reverse aging at the cellular level.

We'll look more deeply into the expanding science of telomeres in chapter 11, but for now it's helpful to visualize two things: Telomeres are like bumpers or tips at the end of shoelaces; they help keep new DNA intact as DNA cells continually divide and replicate into healthy new cells. But as telomeres become shorter and less effective over time, the damage turns them into nefarious actors, degraded molecular structures that can cause or accelerate inflammation, genetic instability, and diseases of aging.

Triathlon Results

As we saw, Joe's triathlon time improved by twenty-four minutes, or 9 percent, in the less than three months before and after his fifty hyperbaric sessions. Gains in his aerobic and anerobic thresholds of 7 percent and 15 percent, respectively, helped turbocharge his power and efficiency.

The triathlon spanned a 0.8-kilometer swim, a 32-kilometer bike race, and a 10-kilometer run. The following table contrasts his results in the swimming, cycling, and running segments.

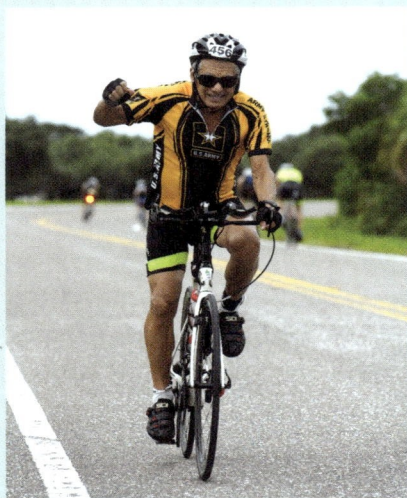

Dr. Joe Maroon, at age eighty-one, cycling in a triathlon after nearly twelve weeks of hyperbarics and related treatments. Time: twenty-four minutes faster than his previous race.

	July 2021 Race	September 2021 Race	Time Change	Relative Change
Total time	3:42:15	3:17:42	-24:33	**-11.0%**
Bike	1:25:45	1:15:22	-10:23	**-12.3%**
Run	1:30:39	1:25:51	-4:48	**-5.5%**
Swim	36:30	27:08	-9:22	**-25.4%**

Figure 2-4: Data in the second column from the right show how much faster Joe completed the full triathlon and each of its three races after completing fifty HBOT sessions. The far-right column shows these gains in percentages.

He emphasized that when medical scientists pay close attention to the details of only one patient case, they can discover important insights. He often cites this one from a 1970s chair of neurosurgery at Harvard Medical School, William Sweet, MD: "We need to establish faith and the capacity of the biologist to reach a valid novel conception on the basis of one single set of facts. There is a staggering difference between zero and one when the one is a good idea."

I strongly agree. I advise my medical colleagues and students to pay attention to patient situations that aren't supposed to happen. These outliers can lead to important discoveries. This is how I first became interested in hyperbaric oxygen therapy, by observing post-stroke diabetic patients being treated in the hyperbarics unit of my hospital who inexplicably regained the ability to walk.

I had to wrestle with what I had casually witnessed: These post-stroke patients were *walking.* As we saw in the first chapter, I was mystified. *How could that be? Why? That isn't supposed to happen.* The resulting clinical study I organized not only changed my attitude about hyperbaric oxygen therapy and its potential. It led me into this largely overlooked new field of medical science, a story so unexpected and life-changing for me that I'll recount it further in chapter 5.

Joe did point out three limitations of his single-subject self-analysis in the scientific paper. One is that additional studies of a larger group of later-age athletes clearly are needed to establish whether his results could be replicated on a large scale. Next, improvements in his triathlon results could have been impacted by factors unrelated to the treatments; to wit, his perception of "full exertion to exhaustion" in both events could have been affected by differences in his rest and diet in the days before both competitions, although he writes that he made no changes in those parameters.

He also noted that it was not known how long the cellular changes during HBOT—biochemical responses producing more stem cells, mitochondria and new blood vessels—will last. Our more recent studies do show that these cellular changes will return to "normal" a few weeks after a client's last session in the hyperbaric chamber.

However, benefits in brain functionality and physical performance resulting from tissue we repair through the sixty sessions in the chamber will continue to increase for another six months, then hold possibly for many years, for brain injuries such as stroke, concussion, PTSD, and Long COVID.

The rate at which a client ages biologically after treatment will vary depending on their fitness routines, diet, and other essential elements for healthy aging. For clients who don't smoke and are not diabetic, new levels of health and performance related to stem cell proliferation, senescent cell reduction, and lengthening of telomeres after treatment can hold for two years or more.

Joe has a plan to avoid or reduce the decline: book twenty daily sessions in an HBOT chamber every eighteen months or two years. He completed his first refresher set in the summer of 2023. By early 2024 he had increased his total chamber sessions to nearly 100. As we'll see in chapter 13, my own practice is to complete a full sixty-session treatment every two years, and between these full treatments book a single chamber session once or twice a week.

HBOT Treatments and Middle-Aged Athletes

We had seen from our work with Alon Day and other elite athletes that HBOT and client-specific treatments in enhanced medicine can significantly elevate the competitive performance of superior athletes in their twenties and thirties. After documenting Alon's improvement, we wondered, *Can HBOT treatments also generate a surge in mitochondria and other elements for regeneration in healthy, middle-aged athletes similar to what top professionals achieve?*

Our clinical study tracking forty master athletes was published in 2022.[10] In addition to mitochondria, we looked to confirm that steep drops in oxygen would produce additional biochemical ingredients—all vital for building a larger capacity for higher athletic performance. We would manage the steep drops by fluctuating oxygen levels for the test group between 1,700 millimeters of mercury per minute (hyperoxic, or high oxygen, level) and 120 millimeters of mercury per minute (normal oxygen level).

In daily HBOT sessions, we repeatedly raised the oxygen levels in air they breathed to 100 percent for twenty minutes, then dropped oxygen levels to normal (21 percent) for five-minute breaks. These fluctuations generated the hyperoxic–hypoxic paradox (HHP), which, in turn, produced hypoxia-inducible factor or HIF (pronounced *heef*).

The test group members' physiology responded as intended with a battery of life-saving defenses designed by nature to counter oxygen deprivation: stem cell proliferations, accelerating mitochondria production, and new blood vessel creation and blood vessel regeneration needed to carry stem cells and mitochondria to vital organs and other tissues.

Moreover, for the first time in humans, we were able to demonstrate *that by generating more HIF,* HBOT improved mitochondria's efficiency in converting oxygen to energy.

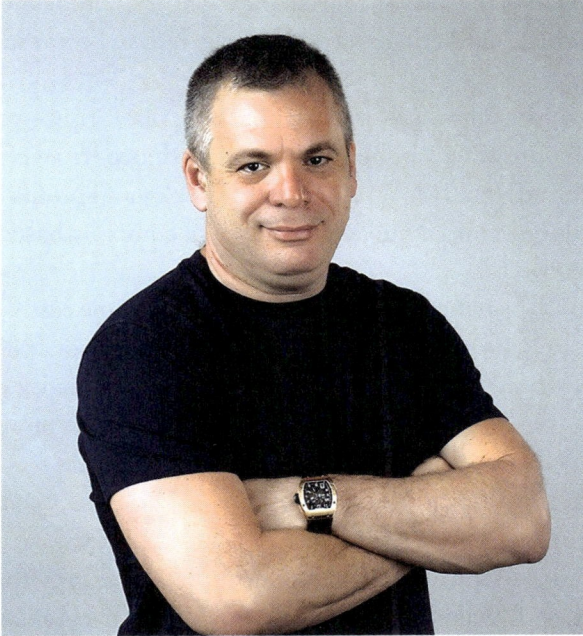

Avishai Abrahami: Digital Visionary, Wix.com Co-Founder, and CEO

In 2006, when he was in his mid-thirties and already a gifted serial entrepreneur, Avishai Abrahami and a colleague co-founded what was to become today's pace-setting website builder, Wix.com.

The long-term vision he and his friend sketched for the company in small-café brainstorms had two parts: One, create digital tools for individuals or small business owners with no coding experience to create inexpensive web pages; that is, their own publishing platforms on their own websites.

The second part was to create tools for professional developers to design software that would give businesses of any size options to add more functions onto these publishing platforms. Multiple functions beyond text and graphics such as digital security, compliance, human resources, sales, marketing and advertising, internal communications, and more.

Yet the free offerings for self-publishing platforms—part one of the vision—proved so popular so quickly that part two became a dream deferred. In 2013, Wix rode surging sales and profits to register one of the largest initial public offerings of a company based in Israel: $725 million.

"It would be tempting to think that success came easily and naturally, the outcome of a secret business formula and not endless hours of tedious work," he wrote at the time.[11] "But the reality is that the early days were more like treading a minefield of potential catastrophes, each equally capable of sinking the Wix vision."

Managing that burst of growth—building the organization, recruiting and developing talent, and pushing hard for continual product innovation—consumed most of his time and energy for the next several years. It was only in the past few years that Avishai and his team were able to introduce new Wix products for program developers—essentially, unveiling part two sixteen years after first conceiving the vision for Wix.

He is one of several exceptional business owners and executives we have helped to recover or bolster their mental and physical capacities. They come to us with a wide range of objectives. What I find so inspiring about these remarkably successful men and women is that they want to go further, to improve their capacities and push higher regardless of what they already have achieved.

Avishai was generous in sharing his story for this chapter.

He was skeptical about HBOT when in 2019 a friend mentioned he was taking the treatment in Tel Aviv. "Why the difference between oxygen at one atmosphere and two? It didn't make sense to me," he says.

A voracious reader in technical and business fields and far beyond, Avishai studied our scientific papers intensively, more so than anyone I had ever met. He encouraged his father, then seventy-two years old, to pursue the full three months' protocol.

"My father was super smart but getting slower, sometimes falling asleep in conversations," Avishai recalls. "After the treatments, he was as fast mentally as he was when he was much younger. His skin looked younger. He got very creative again. That was very interesting to me."

A year later, during COVID lockdowns and global economic upheaval, Avishai decided to schedule the full HBOT program for himself. He had the time, unexpectedly. His crowded schedule of planned international travel had vanished. The crosstown drive to our clinic now was only twenty minutes absent normal Tel Aviv traffic.

We met the first time before his pre-treatment assessments, just before his fiftieth birthday. Talking with Avishai was fascinating, like speaking with an elite neurobiologist. I was amazed. We discussed our methodology for two hours, the pros and cons. Why did we do this, and not that? How does HBOT change the body's biochemistry? How do we measure and evaluate the changes? Why this kind of MRI scan and not that kind of MRI?

He had read exhaustively about HBOT studies by other scientists, articles related to brain degeneration and performance. He remembered the percentage changes in before-and-after treatment metrics. He suggested additional studies to me. It was one of the most interesting biological discussions I ever had—and I did it with the CEO of a computer software company.

Our preliminary neurological analysis put Avishai's cognitive abilities in the top 1 percent. He scored so high we substituted a mix of different tests to gauge his brilliance.

Avishai's Fitness Data		
	Before HBOT	After HBOT
VO_2 (AT)	797	903
VO_2 Max	1433	1831
VO_2/Kg	16.5	20.3
VO_2/HR	11.9	15.1
Watt AT	33	50
Watt Max	109	141

VO_2(AT)—maximal oxygen consumption at the anerobic threshold
VO_2 Max—maximal oxygen capacity
VO_2/Kg—oxygen consumption per weight
Watt AT—maximal power (watt) at the anaerobic threshold
Watt Max—maximal power

Figure 2-5: To illustrate one set of Avishai's evaluation data for fitness, this figure shows results from his cardiopulmonary exercise (treadmill) tests. The left column shows data before HBOT, and the right (with higher numbers) shows his improvement after HBOT.

A burly man with a bearlike torso, Avishai had practiced the Japanese martial arts of ninjutsu since he was a teenager with such focus that he ultimately earned a black belt. Two of ninjutsu's foundational principles are:

1. Always push your abilities.
2. No shortcuts.

In the first month of his HBOT sessions, "I felt more tired than I could ever remember," he recalls. We assured him that this extreme fatigue was a favorable sign, given his brain's high level of metabolic activity.

"Then suddenly, boom. I was full of energy, happier," he says emphatically, with a touch of amazement. "When you train in martial arts at my age, you will rest the next day or two before training again. Now I didn't need those extra days. I didn't need to rest and recover after a workout. Every day, I kept growing. I could finish something, go back in three hours, and do it again. In martial arts fights, I was stronger. I felt like I was eighteen again. I was going to a higher level mentally as well as physically."

A devotee for years of the bestselling video game series *Call of Duty*, Avishai considered himself a top competitor. He gradually realized after the treatments that he was routinely winning most games he entered.

"My information processing speed . . . my decision-making process . . . now was much faster. A massive difference. I was averaging twenty kills and ten deaths before. Now the gap was enormous: twenty-seven kills and only four deaths. My friends wondered what was going on." His new rating in nearly all games: number one in his squad.

Avishai's post-HBOT data for telomeres showed one of the biggest gains we had yet recorded. As the before–after images for Avishai show (Figure 2-6; next page), the average percentage increase of his telomere length was—at 46.8 percent—*twice* the average increase we've observed of 20 to 25 percent.

Avishai's goal was to move faster and more skillfully to expand Wix offerings for professional website developers while continuing to build leadership momentum in the do-it-yourself market.

"I am making more decisions that carry a huge influence on our company's future," he says. "I have to push my boundaries. I am always engaging with super smart people. I have to analyze what they say," he says.

"I know the science here is solid; it's very hard to argue with it anymore. I wanted to become more efficient with my life. The

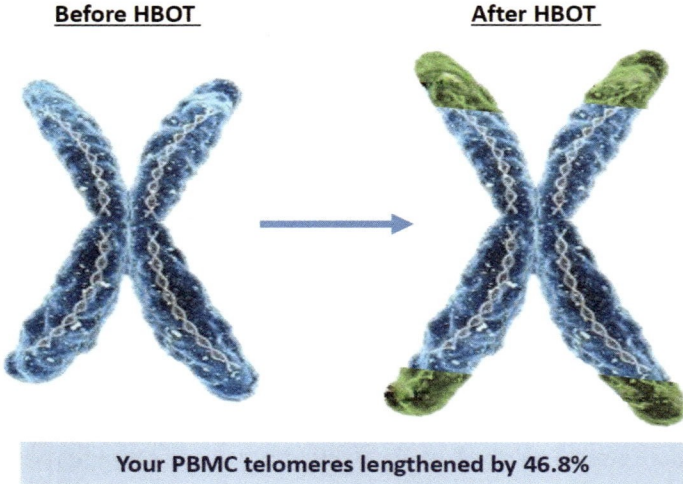

Your average telomeres' length are presented as a percentage change comparing them pre and post HBOT:

Before HBOT   After HBOT

Your PBMC telomeres lengthened by 46.8%

Figure 2-6

treatments gave me an edge I was lacking. I still have that edge and after three years still enjoy the benefits."

Dylan Hartley: A UK Rugby Star's "Near Complete" Recovery

Dylan Hartley was one of England's most famous rugby stars—captain of the national team, winning multiple international trophies—before retiring in 2019 at age thirty-three. When he was hired three years later to coach a local club in Dubai, multiple injuries from his celebrated career had grown worse. "I went to bed every night thinking, *Am I going to get early-onset dementia?*" Married with two young children, Dylan wanted to reclaim his physical and brain health.

Rugby is a full-contact sport with little or no protective headgear, notorious for high-speed collisions and bruising tackles. Dylan played the game competitively at high levels since he was a teenager in New Zealand.

By the time he walked off the pitch after his final match, Dylan had suffered at least twenty documented concussions in competitions and practices, plus many unclassified head injuries that were not flagged as concussions. "I retired because of a left knee injury, but after seventeen years of rugby, I was broken."

He worried over the next few years that he was only marking time before being diagnosed with permanent brain illness. He limped with pain from a degenerative right hip. He dropped things, couldn't abide loud noises, struggled with dizziness, and began to stutter. He couldn't cycle a bike. He couldn't lift a foot to tie his shoelaces. He often was irritable.

As Dylan knew, early-onset dementia indeed was the diagnosis for a former all-star teammate, Steve Thompson. Both were famed, and feared by opponents, for their aggressive style of play, and both had anchored the same position for the Northampton Saints club and England's national team. Thompson retired in 2011.

Dylan moved to the United Arab Republic in 2022 to coach a Dubai rugby club. He became intrigued with HBOT and the other Aviv protocols after the head of physical performance at our Dubai Clinic, Dr. Taif Al Delamie—a former rugby player himself—encouraged Dylan to investigate.

Dylan's continuing worries about early-onset dementia were not misplaced. Our diagnosis would show that he had post-concussion syndrome, the toll from those multiple traumatic brain injuries. His cognitive, physical, and emotional well-being all were in decline and eroding his quality of life.

"I was aware of hyperbaric therapy but had never seen it on the scale that it is here in terms of an all-encompassing program," Dylan says. "I had access to the hyperbaric oxygen. I had access to a dietician, a physio-rehab specialist. I was really motivated to make the most of the opportunity. I didn't want to miss a chance."

Dylan's condition improved markedly—a "near complete" recovery—after he finished his three months of sixty hyperbaric chamber treatments and supporting programs in the spring of 2023. "The metrics, data, and reports from my before–after scans and tests blew me away," he says.

Here is our near-verbatim medical summary of those scans and tests, the type of detailed, science-based readout all clients receive after treatment. Comparing the pre- and post-treatment brain MRI imaging, we found these changes:

1. Increased brain perfusion in multiple cognitive domains, ranging from 10 percent to 43.5 percent in areas related to spatial memory, directionality, sense of smell, memory encoding and retrieval, visuo-motor coordination, hearing processing and language, as measured by the perfusion MRI.

2. Significant improvement in fractional anisotropy, which reflects integrity, directionality, and order of white matter (neuroplasticity), ranging from 5.91 to 20.57 percent in areas related to learning, memory, behavior, sensation, perception, visual processing, learning and formation of new memories, decision-making and cognitive processing of visual information, episodic memory,

language and social–emotional processing, and refinement of motor function, as measured by MRI-DTI.

3. Significant improvement in mean diffusivity (MD), which reflects white matter fiber density, ranging from 4.21 to 11.59 percent in areas related to coordination of arm and leg, learning and formation of new memories, refinement of motor function, processing of visual information, episodic memory, language and social–emotional processing, visual memory, face recognition, and sensory pathway, as measured by MRI-DTI.

In Dylan's pre- and post-SPECT images, we documented these changes:

1. Increased activity in parietal and temporal areas of his brain, ranging from 10 to 18.82 percent.
2. Improvement in related face recognition, word meaning (reading), attention, spatial memory, directionality, somatosensory integration, visuo-motor coordination, memory and control networks, language perception and processing, and memory.

Clinically, we noted these improvements in his cognitive performance:

1. Delayed verbal memory
2. Multitasking
3. Cognitive flexibility and endurance
4. Attention with less distractibility
5. Information processing speed

This indicated that Dylan should have better ability to code, store, and recover verbal information and to understand and react quickly to changes in his environment—what he sees, hears, and experiences physically.

Dylan told us he was better able to focus during meetings and conversations. He had more clarity in his thinking and decision-making. He was able to get more done in shorter periods of time. His irritation with noises faded away.

Our Dubai clinic team concluded that Dylan's scores after the three months "proved favorable for a near complete resolution of his pretreatment symptoms." Moreover, the tests showed "significant improvements in both cognitive and physical parameters."

Dr. Al Delamie used similar qualitative methods to assess Dylan's progress in regaining strength and flexibility: "It was great to lift him up to where he should be."

To back up briefly, let's review the repair and regeneration protocol we tailored for Dylan.

We had started with a comprehensive medical assessment over three days, as we do with every client. The medical history covered his multiple concussions and injuries as a player, his medications during that time and subsequently, and a physician's exam to assess his physical condition. A SPECT brain scan showed lower metabolism, a clear indication of concussion symptoms. We could see the degree of brain damage in his post-concussion syndrome.

We also had Dylan complete MRIs of his physiology so we could pick up on specific issues in his joints and muscles.

A treadmill test of his VO_2 Max showed he had maintained the extraordinarily high cardiovascular performance we often see among professional athletes. Our dietician and nutritionist assessed his body mass index and suggested changes to improve his diet with a strict set of guidelines and get him closer to where we could build his health and performance to what we thought he could and was motivated to achieve.

"I enjoyed this first phase because I learned a lot about myself," Dylan recalls. "I understood what I needed to work on. The only daunting thing was the brain scans. I was very scared to do this . . . to see the truth . . . my reality. As soon as I understood where I was, though, I got very excited. I had the world's best facility at my fingertips to improve myself."

"To have two hours every day to focus on repairing my brain was amazing. I got to target specific areas where I was lacking something, or was low on my scores and other pre-assessments, with different mental challenges they designed for me on the iPad. I saw it as my gym for the brain that got more challenging progressively. My improvement was significant in those areas . . . mind-blowing in many ways."

In our research, we always try to push the boundaries of human limits further. It could be a brain injury patient whose goal is simply to move a finger, an amazing achievement. Or, for people already functioning at an elite level, we want to help push their physiology higher.

In Dylan's case, we were able to help this one-time elite athlete reclaim his mental abilities, avoid lapsing into early-onset dementia, and rebuild a strong foundation in personal fitness. All these delivered a remarkable improvement in his quality of life.

"I wasted three years of my family's life and my life waiting to get something done for my body. The same with my brain. Three years of sleepless nights. Three years of concerns. I know deep within myself that I am better now. I am back doing what I should be doing as a thirty-seven-year-old father. I am in a good place now, which is fantastic."

We believe any career athlete in a full-contact sport such as rugby and American football should seriously consider—before retiring— the HBOT protocol Dylan completed. Multiple traumatic brain

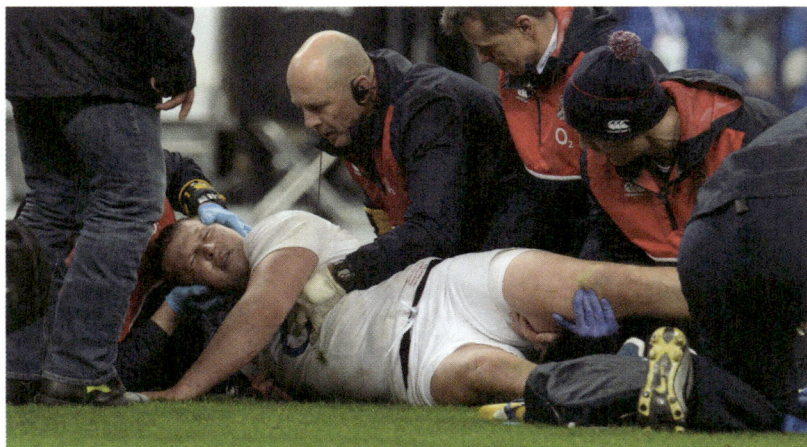

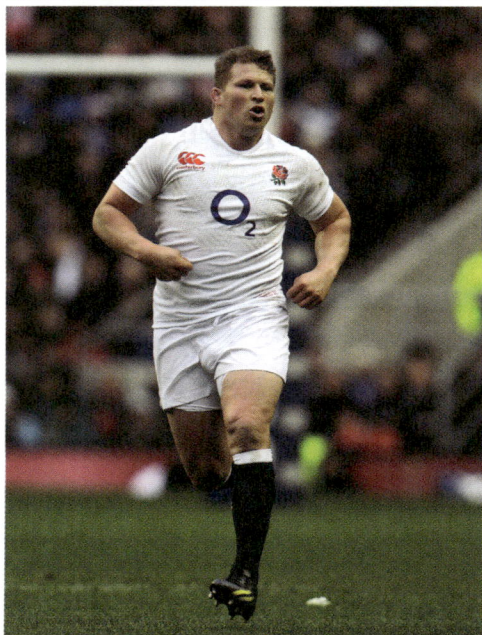

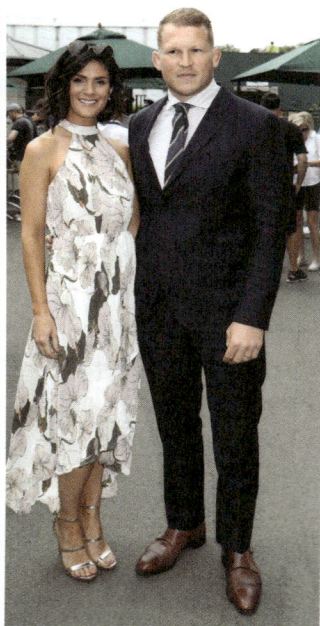

Dylan Hartley in action for England versus Italy in the 2013 RBS 6 Nations tournament (above left), after suffering a severe head injury versus France in the 2016 RBS 6 Nations (top), and with wife Joanne (above right) at the 2019 Wimbledon Tennis Championships a few months before officially announcing his retirement.

injuries may be concussions initially that worsen into chronic traumatic brain injuries.

These more severe injuries may lead to persistent cognitive, emotional, and neurological problems. Our goal is to help elite athletes' minds and bodies recover (to rehabilitate) from damage their sports can cause and reduce risks of brain damage leading to early cognitive decline (prevention).

"You can't be a good sportsman, you can't be a good businessman or husband if your health is poor," he says. "You may be able to get away with it for a while, but it will catch up to you. Everything else around you will start to decline. Don't wait to get better. It might be too late."

. . .

Alon Day, Dr. Joe Maroon, Avishai Abrahami, and Dylan Hartley remind us that we can enhance our physical and mental capacities and achieve more, regardless of what we have already accomplished or what injuries we have sustained. But to do that, it is not enough to be fully dedicated.

We must take advantage of new insights from the scientific world, especially our understanding of how the body works at the cellular level. We need to go beyond the goals of traditional medicine. We need to go beyond the average, to enhance. When we commit through hard work and scientific insights to pushing our capacities higher, there is no limit to what we *homo sapiens* can achieve.

PART II

HOW ENHANCED
MEDICINE WORKS

CHAPTER 3

Fooling Our Bodies into Improving Themselves

My colleagues and I realized some twenty years ago that by applying new ways to design and manage pressure and oxygen concentration, we could accomplish three things: (1) accelerate the growth of stem cells; (2) induce generation of new blood vessels; and (3) improve metabolism in cells to repair damaged tissue that otherwise would not heal.

Those three elements also are fundamental to growing new tissue. They can enhance your performance regardless of your physical condition; it does not matter if you are quadriplegic, average for your age, or a world-class athlete.

A Cascade of Biological Events

In this chapter, we'll look more closely at how the new protocol for HBOT that we use in enhanced medicine—fluctuations in air pressure and oxygen concentration—changes the "normal" environment for the body and how the human body's biochemistry responds and adjusts. When managed professionally, these fluctuations induce physiological changes that repair and regenerate tissue. However, the changes can cause unwanted side effects when not carefully managed by professionals with expertise in this field; this is an important point we'll return to later.

When we as trained physicians treat a patient, we often prescribe a medication that targets a specific enzyme or receptor. We have a very precise goal in mind, such as reducing fever or pain. The same is true in how we have adapted pressure and oxygen concentration for enhanced medicine. By alternating periods of inhaling pure oxygen at high pressure with breathing normal air in a hyperbaric oxygen chamber, we create a cascade of biological events, a set of response–adjustment reactions that repair and regenerate damaged tissue. This is the basis for the new HBOT treatments we apply in enhanced medicine.

Consider exercise as an example of adjustment reactions. When you exercise properly, you stimulate biomechanical activity in cells that delivers more vibrant muscles, blood vessels, heart and lung functions, and more. Or, when you hike or climb in high altitudes, the body adjusts by producing more red blood cells, pumping more blood to circulate oxygen in the red blood cells, and so on. Broadly speaking, these adjustments are triggered when something in the body's environment changes, which is a reflex known medically as *response–reaction.*

To make changes in our remarkably complex human physiology and biology, we must understand the physiology and biology in a very precise, deep way. Once we understand those complexities, which is the work of medical science, we can play around with them. And we can improve them.

Physicians trained in two medical fields that regularly incorporate hyperbarics—diving medicine and emergency medicine—are concerned with treating acute life- or organ-threatening conditions, not repairing and regenerating tissue.

Take, for example, "the bends." Decompression sickness develops in divers if air bubbles prevent oxygen from reaching tissue, an affliction caused by rising too rapidly to the surface. The bubbles need to be compressed to permit oxygen flows to recover, which is why we move divers into a hyperbaric chamber quickly once symptoms such as headache, joint pain, confusion, and other neurological symptoms accumulate after they have surfaced too rapidly. The elevated pressure in the chamber shrinks the air bubbles, which is necessary for the diver's biology to recalibrate to lighter air pressure above water.

In emergency medicine, the threat to a patient's organs or life is usually related to a lack of oxygen. Carbon monoxide intoxication can block oxygen flows in red blood cells as carbon monoxide molecules bind to hemoglobin, essentially competing with oxygen to be transported in the bloodstream. (Patients rescued from fires arriving in emergency rooms frequently have inhaled dangerous carbon monoxide gases.) A hyperbaric chamber enables us to increase blood oxygenation rapidly.

Typically, one to three sessions in a hyperbaric chamber are enough to cure acute conditions such as these that we see in diving and emergency medicine.

Perceived Lack of Oxygen Is the Trigger for Repair and Regeneration

During a typical two-hour HBOT session in the hyperbaric chamber, the pressure in arteries rises to around 1,520 millimeters of mercury, some fifteen times the normal pressure at sea level, or 120 millimeters of mercury. Meanwhile, clients breathe pure oxygen through a mask, which is absorbed nearly fifteen times more than the normal amount of oxygen breathed at sea level. During that time, the amount of dissolved oxygen generated is sufficient for all the body's energy demand because oxygen in these conditions can be delivered through blood flows or between tissues to locations red blood cells cannot reach.

While still in the chamber, clients remove the oxygen mask at three intervals for brief periods (five minutes) when they breathe normal air with the pressure still twice that at sea level, abbreviated as 2 ATA for two atmospheres absolute. Oxygen concentration drops sharply during these breaks from very high to slightly high. These repeated fluctuations, in addition to daily gaps between sessions, are interpreted at the cellular level as a lack of oxygen (hypoxia) even though actual oxygen levels are higher than normal (hyperoxia).

As we will see shortly, the body's perceived lack of oxygen is the trigger for tissue repair and regeneration in a hyper-oxygenized (hyperoxic) environment.

The fact that oxygen is necessary to sustain life in animals, including humans, has been a cornerstone of modern biology for two centuries. Going back 800 million years, oxygen has been the most essential biological foundation for life on Earth, enabling animal and then human life to evolve from single-cell organisms.

Oxygen in the blood can be in one of two compartments. Dissolved oxygen is in blood plasma, the liquid of the bloodstream, in contrast to oxygen in hemoglobin, the protein of red blood cells that transports oxygen. At sea level, when we breathe normal air with 21 percent oxygen, the separation of oxygen into red blood cells and plasma occurs naturally. Hyperbaric chamber treatments affect only dissolved oxygen in plasma.

The volume of red blood cells determines how much oxygen is being delivered to cells. Under normal conditions, red blood cells are the dominant transport means for oxygen, because most oxygen is carried in hemoglobin. The amount of dissolved oxygen in blood varies. Under normal conditions, it is negligible, about 2 percent of total oxygen in the bloodstream. (We normally have 10 to 20 grams of hemoglobin in every 100 millimeters of blood.)

Not so when pure oxygen is breathed at elevated pressures of 2 ATA or higher. The amount of dissolved oxygen soars to levels where the oxygen supply can meet *all* energy demand in the body. And this brings us to a distinctive principle in HBOT treatments: **oxygen can be delivered to and even bypass small arteries with blockages to reach tissues and cells that red blood cells cannot reach due to those blockages.**

How Dissolved Oxygen Helps to Heal

Dissolved oxygen is effective in reaching and healing wounds that could not be healed otherwise due to reduced (ischemic) blood flow.

Both oxygen and pressure-sensitive genes that are especially common in smooth muscle are targeted by dissolved oxygen to improve mitochondria metabolism and proliferation, stem cell proliferation and migration, and angiogenesis factors.

The healing properties of dissolved oxygen are not limited to a specific organ or wound. Rather, they are sensed in multiple organs, including the brain and heart.

Collectively, these benefits are broadly essential for regenerating tissue. Wounds cannot heal and tissue cannot be repaired without sufficient oxygen supply.

Throughout much of the late twentieth century, hyperbarics were used to treat wounds that could not heal because of insufficient oxygen supplies linked to damage in blood vessels. (These are known as *ischemic wounds.*) Blood flows in small arteries were inhibited. HBOT was used to treat common ischemic nonhealing wounds, most often diabetic wounds and tissue damage caused by radiation therapy for cancer patients. Diabetics typically have narrowing blood vessel passages (atherosclerosis) that culminate in poor circulation and oxygen supply. Radiation treatments designed to kill cancer cells may also damage small blood vessels in healthy tissues surrounding targeted tumors.

Calibrating Fluctuations in Oxygen and Air Pressure

Many discoveries over the past two decades have shown how hyperbaric medicine can go beyond healing ischemic wounds to regenerate tissue. In essence, we learned how to calibrate fluctuations in oxygen levels and pressure to induce regenerative processes that heal damaged tissues and generate healthy new tissues.

The combined action of both hyperoxia (high oxygen conditions) and hyperbaric pressure (2 ATA or more) has a significant impact in addition to tissue oxygenation. Targeting oxygen and pressure-sensitive genes improves chemical processes (metabolism) of mitochondria and accelerates mitochondria production; stimulates more rapid production of stem cells and speeds their distribution to where they are needed; and induces growth of new blood vessels (angiogenesis) and better blood flow in ischemic areas.

None of these benefits is limited to a specific organ or wound. Rather, cells in multiple organs can sense and respond to these biochemical changes. This includes in the brain, where for years I and my teams have focused much of our research. As we will explore in Part II, we have identified brain injuries caused by several neurological disorders that the new HBOT protocol heals, including stroke, concussion, fibromyalgia, post-traumatic stress disorder (PTSD), and Long COVID. (What about Alzheimer's disease? I'm asked about this frequently. We don't know, but we are investigating. Our clinical investigations on whether HBOT can slow or reverse damage in early Alzheimer's began in 2023.) In separate chapters, we will look closely at how we came to diagnose and treat each of these disorders.

As we saw in chapter 1, sparking higher levels of the body's production of the hypoxia-inducible factor, or HIF (pronounced *heef*), specifically the protein HIF-1 alpha, is a core objective of the molecular biology foundations in HBOT treatments. The intermittent increase of oxygen concentration during chamber sessions mimics hypoxia (low oxygen conditions). The fluctuations initiate signals from proteins for gene expression (mediators) and cellular responses that arise when the body senses dangerous oxygen deprivation. Yet, in professionally managed HBOT, there are no life-threatening dangers. This is the *hyperoxic–hypoxic paradox,* or HHP.

Intermittent exposure to pure oxygen (hyperoxic) during HBOT sessions is designed to trigger biochemical responses in cells for a virtuous regenerative cascade in tissues: increasing levels of HIF-1, activity of matrix metalloproteinases (MMP), levels of vascular endothelial growth factor (VEG-F), stem cell proliferation, and levels of factors that generate new blood vessel growth (angiogenesis). New blood vessels help improve blood flows to low-oxygen or oxygen-deprived (ischemic) tissue. HBOT treatments also improve circulation of specific cells (endothelial progenitor cells—EPCs) that restore the lining of blood vessels after a sudden, often severe injury (acute insult), such as a broken bone.

Flashpoint for Survival Alarm System

Cells sense a survival threat from the perceived low-oxygen condition, even though the body actually is in a high-oxygen environment. That's the paradox. The cells respond this way because waves of HIF that normally arise in severe oxygen-deprived situations (hypoxia) are pouring into cell nuclei.

HIF is the flashpoint of an alarm system that sets in motion a full cascade of genes necessary to accelerate oxygen production and delivery and create more energy. A protein, HIF initiates the expression of certain parts of the DNA into RNA, further generating active proteins that trigger several aspects of this cascade. As we will see, HIF is one of the most vital—and recent—biochemical insights in enhanced medicine. It has an important role in the regeneration and maintenance of essential organs that are highly dependent on oxygen, such as the brain and the heart.

My term for these manifold physiological and biological enhancements is *hyperoxic synchronized environment*. All these elements need to work together harmoniously and at the same time to produce this surge in HIF, just like a garden needs the right combination of nutrients and water for a new plant to take root, grow, and thrive.

In high-oxygen conditions (hyperoxia), HIF actually breaks down and the expression of those genes is inhibited because the body has no need for the surge in oxygen activity its presence normally triggers. The full cascade of genetic signals that HIF contributes to restart metabolic adaptation and cellular revival is shut down.

This sleight of hand—convincing the body in normal conditions that it needs a surge of oxygen—is an example of what I was referring to a few pages back when I said that once we understand the complexities of physiology and biology in a very precise way, we can play around with it and improve it. This is what we are doing with the new protocol for HBOT, sparking a surge of HIF through the microbiology of the hyperoxic–hypoxic paradox (see Figure 3-1).

Bring on the Scavengers

This next point may strike you as counterintuitive. The absolute value of oxygen in the chamber—whether low, high, or normal—is not what determines the expression or breaking down of HIF-1a. It is the balance that cells sense between unstable molecules that can damage DNA, RNA, and proteins if too abundant, and extraordinary cell proteins whose job is to eliminate those unstable molecules by binding and neutralizing those molecules. The unstable molecules are known as *reactive oxygen species*, or RO. These are the eliminating proteins, the scavengers.

In a lone event of high-oxygen exposure (hyperoxia), such as a single session in the hyperbaric chamber, the normal balance between scavengers and ROS tilts ominously toward favoring the unstable molecules. That balance is always dynamic. Why? Reactive oxygen species are generated and eliminated rapidly, within seconds or minutes. Because scavengers are proteins, they take longer to produce and, once created, can stay active in "eating" ROS for days or weeks. In effect, in a steady state, the volume of ROS fluctuates quickly, and the volume of scavenger proteins does not.

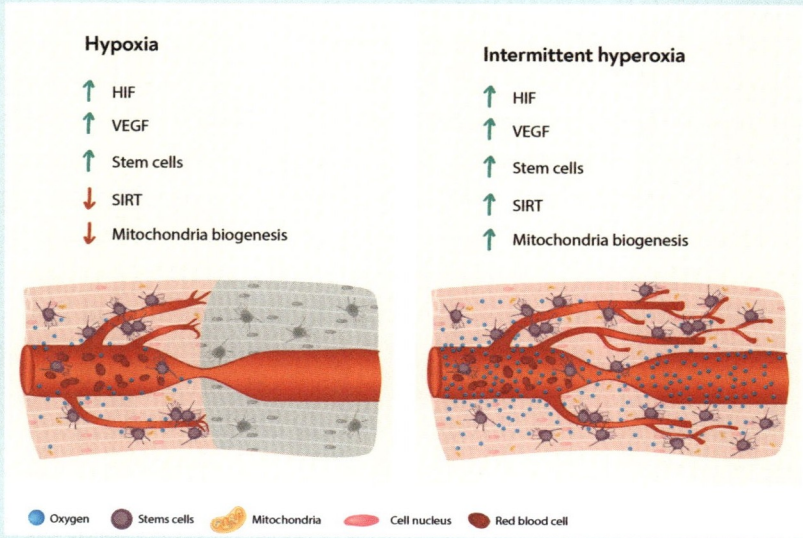

Figure 3-1: The major cellular response cascade initiated by hypoxia and by intermittent hyperoxia.

Hypoxia is the natural trigger for mitochondria-induced metabolic changes via elevated levels of HIF, VEG-F, Sirtuin, mitochondria metabolic changes, SC proliferation, and migration (left image).

Fluctuations in oxygen levels can trigger a cellular cascade that is usually triggered by hypoxia. This intermittent application of abnormally high oxygen levels, or hyperoxia, stimulates tissue regeneration without the hazardous effects of hypoxia—dangerously low levels of oxygen supply. All these cellular processes happen without the hazardous damage related to lack of oxygen supply—a huge benefit. This phenomenon is known as the "hyperoxic–hypoxic paradox" (right image).

Legend: HIF: hypoxic-inducible factor;
VEG-F: vascular endothelial growth factor; SIRT: Sirtuin.

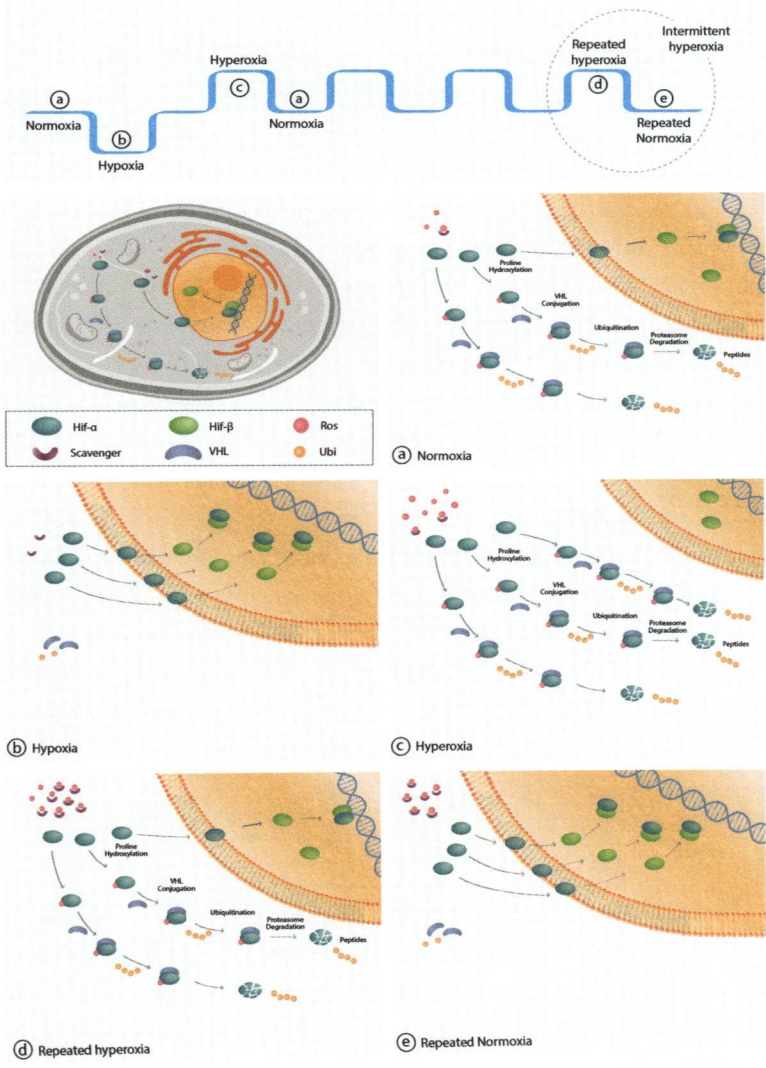

Figure 3-2: The intracellular cascade of HIF-1 alpha.

HIF-1 is a heterodimer, a molecule complex with two different proteins, composed of cytoplasmatic HIF-1α and the nuclear HIF-1β subunits. (a) Under normal oxygen environments, the ratio of ROS/scavenger is high, and the free ROS molecules initiate HIF-1α hydroxylation. HIF-1α subunits become a target for VHLp (von Hippel–Lindau protein) which facilitates degradation, or breakdown, of HIF-1α subunits. (b) Under hypoxic conditions, less oxygen and ROS molecules are available, HIF-1α subunits are not hydrolyzed, and more HIF-1α subunits penetrate the nucleus to conjugate with HIF-1α subunits and generate the active HIF transcription factor; in other words, turning on a key to activate the expression of other genes. (c) In the hyperoxic environment, more ROS and oxygen are available; thus more HIF-1α subunits are hydrolyzed (broken down by water) and degraded. (d) The adaptive response to repeated hyperoxia includes increases in the production of scavengers that adjust to the increased ROS generation. Thus, the ROS/scavenger ratio gradually becomes similar to the ratio under normal oxygen environment prior to initiating repeated hyperoxic exposures. (e) Upon return to normoxia, following repeated hyperoxic exposures, the ratio of ROS/scavenger is low due to the fact scavengers' elimination half-life ($T_{1/2}$) is significantly longer than the $T_{1/2}$ of ROS. Accordingly, less HIF-1α subunits are hydroxylated, and more of them penetrate the nucleus, conjugate with HIF-1α to generate the active HIF, similar to the hypoxic state.

In our HBOT protocols, repeated exposure to high oxygen triggers production of more scavenger proteins because the body perceives the high-oxygen condition as a new steady state. Scavengers predominate in this new steady state. As oxygen levels return to normal, there is a higher level of scavengers as compared with ROS.

It is this sustained dominance of scavenger proteins that makes it easy for HIF-1a to be expressed abundantly as if it were in a low-oxygen environment and for HIF-1a to enter cell nuclei. Once inside cell nuclei, HIF-1a (alpha) bind to HIF-1α (beta) to activate a genetic switch (transcriptor factor) that initiates the virtuous biological cascade: new stem cells, mitochondria, VEG-F, and growth of new blood vessels to deliver more oxygen to where it is needed.

HIF Discovery and, Twenty-Four Years Later, the Nobel Prize

HIF clearly has a major role in the virtuous biological cascade, but we don't know if it is the only one. In biology, generally speaking, there is never one path. What we believe we know now may change over time.

It may take between fifteen and twenty HBOT sessions, or roughly three or four weeks, for HIF's favorable new conditions to take place, but once it does, HIF production continues and is compounded through the rest of the treatment. For another eight or nine weeks, HIF production stimulates more generation of stem cells, mitochondria, VEG-F, and angiogenesis.

We have only understood the role of HIF in how cells detect and react to changing levels of oxygen since it was discovered in 1995 by Gregg Semenza, a physician and medical scientist at Johns Hopkins University. His research with HIF, especially in cancer and cardiovascular disease, soon was further developed by William Kaelin Jr., a physician–scientist at Harvard Medical School and Dana-Farber Cancer Institute, and Sir Peter Ratcliffe, a physician–scientist at Oxford University.[1]

The trio shared the Nobel Prize for Physiology or Medicine in 2019.[2] In its award announcement, the Nobel Committee emphasized that many groups have "shown the robustness of the HIF pathway" since the three scientists' discoveries. The committee further noted that, in addition to cancer and kidney disease, "this discovery of HIF-1 has the potential to result in treatments for diseases such as blood disorders, blinding eye diseases, coronary artery disease, and other conditions." They added that the three laureates have "remained central figures in this work" and "increased our understanding of the physiological roles played by hypoxic response in health and disease."[3]

Our Protocol in the Chamber to Stimulate HIF Production

- Clients inhale pure oxygen through a mask in four twenty-minute sequences at pressures exceeding what is normal at sea level. The most common, scientifically proven protocols for our hyperbaric sessions, or "dives," include breathing 100 percent oxygen at 2 ATA with five-minute air breaks after each twenty-minute session.
- During those five-minute breaks, masks come off and clients often chat or rest as they breathe normal air, which is 21 percent oxygen, at the same elevated pressure of 2 ATA.
- Meanwhile, elevated air pressure pushes the oxygen pressure in arteries to 1,520 millimeters of mercury, or nearly fifteen times the normal level of around 120 millimeters of mercury at sea level.
- After around four weeks of daily repeated sessions, five days per week, the body perceives oxygen levels in a normal room environment as "dangerously" low (hypoxia), yet actual oxygen levels are high, so there is no real danger. This is the hyperoxic–hypoxic paradox, or HHP.
- Our cells perceive that rapid decline from very high oxygen to normal oxygen as a signal that oxygen intake is seriously impaired or *shut down.*

- Our biology responds, producing a protein known as the *hypoxia-inducible factor,* or HIF. This protein, pronounced *heef,* initiates a series of events including the expression of genes and proteins responsible for changes in cellular metabolism that create the regenerative cascade.

We realized from our initial studies that the two-hour sessions in the hyperbaric chamber produced the best biological response when they are repeated five days each week for three months and monitored by medical professionals in the chamber and by experts tracking the sessions in real time at a nearby data center. It totals to sixty sessions in all.

The presence of a medical professional in the chamber is crucial to ensure patient safety, to tightly monitor the pressure (at 2 ATA), the oxygen levels (pure oxygen or normal air at 21 percent oxygen), and the length of time the mask with pure oxygen is on. (The fluctuations between pure oxygen and normal air are more important than the oxygen per se.) Any unanticipated change could make the treatment ineffective.

Our program also includes analyses by neuropsychologists of data generated from a series of cognitive drills assigned during "dive" sessions, drills that Alon Day and Dylan Hartley mentioned in chapter 2. These computer-generated drills, displayed on touch-screen tablets, are calibrated to improve specific skills that clients hope to improve in their own mental agility and acuity, such as sharper attention, memory, and processing speed. As Dylan put it, "I saw it as my gym for the brain that got more challenging progressively."

Physical fitness routines with personal trainers and nutrition plans with professional dieticians also are customized for clients, and progress is monitored. Physicians are available to consult with clients every day about their progress and any concerns, drawing from data and insights circulated regularly among staff professionals.

Treating Toxic Symptoms vs. Enhancing Our Biology

It is gratifying to see more medical professionals and medical scientists advancing the science of HBOT for repairing and regenerating tissue. Many of these physicians were trained in internal medicine, as I was, or physiological neurology (biology of the nervous system). We focus on the body's core biology to stimulate production and proliferation of stem cells and mitochondria and to induce angiogenesis for more efficient perfusion.

Yet, until now, most physicians trained in hyperbarics have had a narrower view. This is because most medical schools teach about HBOT with respect to decompression sickness or medical emergencies, not any of the protocols we use to stimulate regenerative effects through the fluctuations of pressure and oxygen that define HHP. When you open a medical textbook, you do not find anything about the hyperoxic–hypoxic paradox.

What we practice in enhanced medicine is not in the comfort zone of a typical physician. In our clinics, physicians utilizing HHP were trained either in internal medicine, general medicine, or neurology. It is easier to teach physicians from these fields about diving and emergency medicine than vice versa. In effect, we are breaking the old paradigm for how HBOT is used.

Caution: Beware of Charlatans

Many hyperbaric providers have emerged in recent years as the benefits of this medical field have advanced. Some are highly reputable, matching disciplined procedures with desired outcomes, yet there is a lot of inaccurate information and irresponsible sales pitches going around. This has generated some confusion and, inevitably, disappointment about HBOT for too many people.

Many of these hyperbaric centers are uncontrolled, unregulated, and ineffective. Their proprietors are charlatans. Then, too, small hyperbaric "tents" or "tubes" for home use that first appeared decades ago were vastly oversold. Many of these types of products are still on the market, with prices ranging from a few thousand dollars to more than $20,000, despite the fact that they have not proved to be effective.

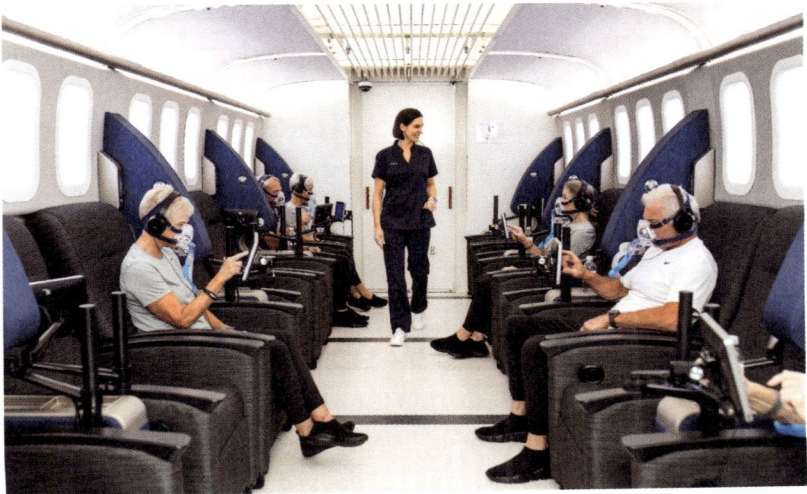

Figure 3-3. Here is what the enhanced medicine standard for hyperbaric oxygen treatments looks like: a medical-grade chamber that is well controlled, regulated, monitored, and supervised by a professional medical team. This one has fourteen seats, seven on each side of the chamber.

Moreover, the tubes are not safe. There is no quality assurance on the air pumped into the tube or sack from the compressor or the rate at which air inside the tube is refreshed. If not refreshed often, the air can be polluted with bacteria, oils, and gases with high concentrations of carbon monoxide (CO) or carbon dioxide (CO_2) that can cause serious damage to lungs and the cardiovascular system. In addition, there is no safety assurance. Tubes have been known to explode, injuring the user and breaking or destroying things nearby.

I've met some physicians who became reflexively dismissive about HBOT after hearing a patient report no medical benefit from sleeping in a hyperbaric "tent" they purchased online from China or other unreliable sources. If that story is all a physician knows about HBOT, of course they will be skeptical. That experience has nothing to do with enhanced medicine.

It's important to emphasize the depth of the science, sophistication, and distinction of the new HBOT protocols and equipment targeting HHP to achieve desired outcomes in enhanced medicine.

I always urge people to be aware that any HBOT treatments they consider should be provided only in medical-grade facilities with quality care assured by a physician, technician, and nurses who are professionals and specialists in this field. Otherwise, you could be receiving something else that has not been proved effective. You could be risking your health.

Vascular Endothelial Growth Factor (VEG-F): Growing and Remodeling Blood Vessels

VEG-F, the vascular endothelial growth factor, is another vital protein in the biological response to HBOT. Its role is to activate growth of new blood vessels (angiogenesis). Angiogenesis opens new pathways for blood flow to bypass narrow or blocked areas in those existing vessels. VEG-F production is triggered as cells produce HIF-1.

In addition, VEG-F stimulates production of cells manufactured in bone marrow that contribute to angiogenesis and then has those cells ferried through the bloodstream to areas where oxygen supply is needed the most, especially in the brain and heart. These are *bone marrow–derived angiogenic cells*, or BMDACs.

These findings and more are part of mounting evidence from patient and animal studies showing that HBOT sessions induce these two crucial elements for angiogenesis—VEG-F and endothelial progenitor cells (EPC). Patient studies confirm that repeated daily HBOT sessions in enhanced medicine raise the circulating levels of VEG-F and EPCs. This improves blood flow in areas where a healthy flow had waned because of a reduced blood supply that resulted in a lack of oxygen and other nutrients.

Sirtuins: Protecting against Disease

Sirtuins are another family of proteins that play a role in cellular metabolism. Their growth and proliferation also are stimulated by repeated HBOT sessions. Some researchers exploring the science of aging, of longevity, have taken a keen interest in sirtuins. Sirtuins are an attractive target for treating disease and promoting tissue regeneration at the cellular level. They are closely linked to the benefits of accelerated mitochondria performance as well as growth and tissue recovery from injury or inflammation. When certain sirtuins are abundant, they help protect against many cancers, type 2 diabetes, and heart disease.

Mitochondria Biogenesis: Delivering More Oxygen

Mitochondria is the part of a cell that generates energy—one of three specialized parts known as *organelles*. (The other two are nuclei, which store genetic information, and ribosomes, which manufacture protein.) Maintaining a steady supply and potency of mitochondria is crucial throughout life.

We have shown in both animal and human studies that the repeated HBOT sessions over three months improves the functioning of mitochondria already present in cells, initiates production of more mitochondria, and increase our heart and lung capacity to deliver more oxygen to muscles; in other words, strengthens our cardiovascular fitness. Whenever you want to build or restore capacity to lift your biological performance, you must invest energy. Oxygen is the mitochondria's basic raw material for producing that energy.

We have natural processes for breaking down and clearing out damaged mitochondria (known as *mitophagy*) and for generating new supplies of smoothly functioning mitochondria. Mitochondria work to divide and grow into new mitochondria, a process known as *mitochondria biogenesis*. Mitochondria biogenesis is crucial to preserve the integrity of most human cells.

We can go further now, thanks to data acquired from multiple studies in recent years, and assert that age-related brain diseases such as mild cognitive impairment, Alzheimer's disease, and Parkinson's disease as well as cardiovascular diseases and cancer may be related to malfunctioning mitochondria.

There is growing evidence that mitochondria also help protect neurons from damage. Recent studies showed that mitochondria can move between cells that keep neurons functioning well to neurons themselves. These cells are known as *astrocytes*. Neurons can release and transfer damaged mitochondria to astrocytes for disposal and recycling. Astrocytes can release healthy mitochondria that enter neurons. One study took another step, demonstrating that the HBOT protocol we use at 2 ATA promotes resilience of neurons more susceptible to inflammation by sending more healthy mitochondria from astrocytes to those neuronal cells.[4] The mitochondria are affected directly by the amount of dissolved oxygen that reaches them by diffusion.

The impact on mitochondria of intermittent changes in oxygen concentration created during HBOT sessions over time is like the intense interval training during fitness workouts that builds maximal aerobic capacity—the amount of oxygen our heart and lungs can process at the peak of any physical activity. Think of runners sprinting short distances repeatedly or cyclists accelerating to maximum speeds. Their goal is to run or cycle faster. They are striving to elevate their maximal aerobic capacity.

The new HBOT protocols help mitochondria proliferate rapidly and function more efficiently in converting oxygen to energy. These protocols generate more blood vessels and enable more blood to flow into capillaries that carry more stem cells and more oxygen to more potent mitochondria.

Stem Cells: Building Stones for Tissue Repair

Stem cells do two remarkable things: They can precisely replicate their biological structures, dividing indefinitely to produce more of the same cell, and they can "print" bespoke three-dimensional repair kits of cells needed to heal damaged tissue. They are building stones for repairing damaged tissue.

Oxygen fluctuations in the new HBOT protocol serve as an electrical charge the printer needs to operate. Mitochondria within stem cells sense, provide, and activate that electrical charge.

Our clinical studies and those of others conducted for more than a decade clearly demonstrate many positive enhancements for stem cell growth and activity. We've established, for instance, how new HBOT protocols trigger three primary groups of stem cells in mammals. One group replenishes blood and immune cells (hematopoietic), another maintains skin cells on the outer surface of the body (basal), and a third maintains cells in bone, cartilage, muscle, and fat cells (mesenchymal).

Among several subgroups with specific roles, stem cells in certain areas of the adult brain generate nerve cells and supporting cells, including astrocytes and another known as *oligodendrocytes*. Stem cells also have many properties that make them an appealing resource for physicians seeking therapies for a variety of disorders.

Most of the time, when the body is healthy and in a steady state, stem cells are dormant, like bears sleeping in winter with very low metabolic requirements. But the hyperoxic–hypoxic paradox induced by new HBOT brings stem cells back to full metabolic activity with a rush. The perceived hypoxia in our body chemistry triggers a surge in stem cell production. New cells migrate to where they are most needed, anywhere in the body, and with greater capacity to "reprint" themselves. That is, stem cells can transform into whatever cells the body signals it needs to maintain or recover a more vibrant biology and accompanying physiological performance.

The main advantage in stirring stem cells from hibernation to surging growth and activity with HBOT protocols is that those hyperbaric chamber sessions induce the body to generate energy safely when the sessions are managed properly by professionals.

As we've seen, oxygen plays an important role in regulating how rapidly stem cells reproduce and move to where they are most needed in the body. The *perceived* low-oxygen condition sparks our biology into initiating more stem cell delivery. The response activates more growth and distribution of VEG-F. That protein then sparks the growth of new blood vessels to carry stem cells and regenerates aging blood vessels to do the same thing but more effectively.

Powerful Therapeutic Tool

Just as Albert Einstein's theory of relativity explored and explained the basic physics of our cosmos, we can explore the same phenomena in the micro-cosmos, the ways in which we interpret and apply the laws of biophysics in our cells.

As we saw in Figure 3-2, all the required elements for the biological cascade to repair and regenerate tissue can be induced by "fooling" how cells interpret these intermittent surges and declines of available oxygen. Again, and I'm repeating here to underscore their importance, these elements include HIF, VEG-F, other metabolic mediators, mitochondrial biogenesis, and stem cell proliferation and migration.

The new protocol of HBOT is a powerful therapeutic tool when applied consistently over three months by professionals in carefully managed hyperbaric chambers. The treatments address multiple types of tissue damage calling for better, faster regeneration. These professionals carefully vet participants to ensure they have no medical conditions, such as lung emphysema with trapped air, inner ear disorders, or active epileptic locos in the brain that would put them at risk during hyperbaric treatments.

Now we're ready to turn to the fascinating cosmos of our own inner space, the human brain. In the next chapters, we will see how combining the hyperoxic–hypoxic paradox with other core principles in enhanced medicine discussed in chapter 1 works to repair the symptoms and damage of diseases that have long been considered beyond hope.

Key Takeaways

1. The goal of HBOT in enhanced medicine is to manage oxygen fluctuations in a pressurized environment to induce physiological changes that repair and regenerate damaged tissue.

2. By alternating periods of inhaling pure oxygen at high pressure with breathing normal air in a hyperbaric

oxygen chamber, we create a cascade of biological events, a set of response–adjustment reactions that repair and regenerate damaged tissue.

3. In the hyperbaric chamber, with 100 percent oxygen pressurized at 2 ATA, dissolved oxygen can be delivered even to locations where red blood cells cannot reach due to occlusions, or blockages, in small arteries.

4. The hypoxic-inducible factor, or HIF, is the flashpoint of an alarm system that sets in motion a full cascade of genes necessary to accelerate oxygen production and delivery and create more energy.

CHAPTER 4

The Brain as a Tissue

The human brain is our inner space—determining who we are and how we perceive the world that surrounds us. It contains an estimated 90 billion neurons, the cells that orchestrate and monitor communications in our body's central nervous system.

If you have ever seen a galaxy photo or peered up at the stars through a telescope, you can imagine the microscopic image of our brain with its dazzling, infinite complexity. Scientists estimate that the Milky Way galaxy may have the same number of stars as we have neurons in our brain.

Neurons become active by passing signals to each other via intricate connections called *synapses*; our brain has an estimated 100 trillion synaptic connections. They transmit the signals in an electrical and chemical network that extends from the more sophisticated neurons in the brain, the cortical pyramidal cells, to neurons, muscles, and organs everywhere else in the body.

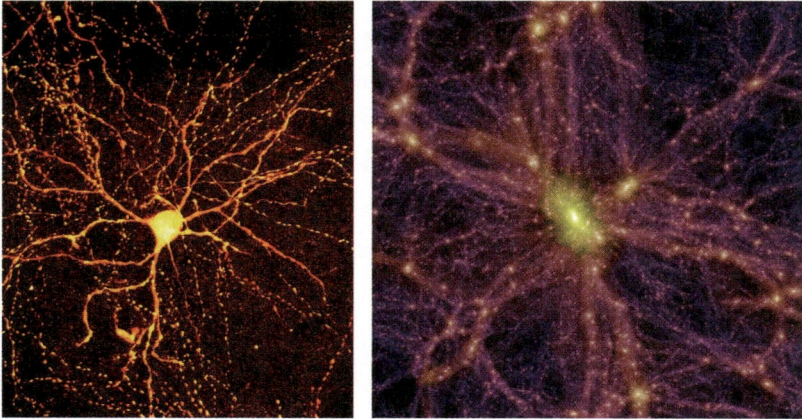

Figure 4-1: LEFT: Brain cell neuron of a bird. RIGHT: Large-scale simulation of the universe.

The outer layer of the brain, the cortex, is the largest and most complex of any species in *homo sapiens* and became our single biggest advantage over all other species on Earth. Our brains could not have developed far beyond other animals today if our predecessors had not learned how to control fire and cook food.

That ingenious step enabled us to divert energy once consumed in digesting raw food to expanding the cortex. Further evolutionary pressures—such as social interactions and organizational activities involved in obtaining the food—led to the development of larger brains. Across the millennia of evolution, *homo sapiens* became rulers of this planet. Our large brain gave us the capacity to think abstractly, to communicate and organize, to imagine and prepare for a better future.

Our superior brains enable us to frame—and answer—basic questions such as: How can we avoid dangers, preserve life, and improve our living conditions? How can we adapt raw materials in the Earth's crust to create and master new technologies?

We, *homo sapiens,* use only 8 to 15 percent of our total energy consumption for digestion, in contrast to most animals, whose digestion burns two times as much and more. Every day, we burn more calories thinking (340 calories, on average) than we do during an hour of light gardening, a leisurely bike ride of forty-five minutes, or running at a pace of ten minutes per mile for half an hour.

Yet, most of us are using only 5 to 10 percent of our maximal brain capacity. The question is, why? Why are we using only a fraction? The answer is that we don't have enough oxygen to fuel more neuron activity. At any given moment, the brain is using all the oxygen available in its blood supply. It must set priorities: to deliver more oxygen to those regions that are essential for the specific task or tasks needed at that moment. The less essential regions at that moment, in effect, are put on standby.

For example, if I am speaking on a mobile phone, more of that oxygen will go to the part of the brain that governs speaking. I might miss a turn as a result because my brain is paying less attention to what I am seeing, delivering less oxygen to the area that governs my visual processing. If I move a hand holding the mobile phone, more oxygen flows to the area of the brain responsible for hand movement.

My main point here is that our brains are oxygen-deprived even under normal healthy conditions. When we have a brain injury, our brains naturally respond by delivering more of the available oxygen to repair the damage in those areas of the brain at the expense of what are now more areas of the brain that—as a result of the injury—have less claim on the available blood supply. It is only logical then that increasing blood flows can improve performance in healthy brains and accelerate healing in injured areas of the brain.

More Oxygen, More Metabolism, More Brain Power

Brain capacity is a major, if not a dominant, factor in how well we prosper relative to others in a given society. Darwin's law predicts that succeeding generations will develop more brain capacity. And that is the case. There has been a threefold increase in brain size in a mere 2.5 million years. With each new generation, remarkable as it may seem, the human cortex continues to expand, leading to ever higher cognitive potential.

My Co-Author for This Chapter, Amir Hadanny

In writing this chapter, I worked closely with my brilliant colleague Amir Hadanny.

Already a neurosurgeon and once one of my top medical students and residents at Shamir Medical Center, Amir later added a PhD in artificial intelligence and data management to his resume.

Amir and I have collaborated on many studies and published papers over the past several years, such as the role of oxygen as a limiting factor in how the brain functions and how HBOT—specifically, the hyperoxic–hypoxic paradox in enhanced medicine—promotes healing for myriad brain injuries. The first article we co-authored in 2015 described the case of a diver suffering from a consistent brain injury from decompression after surfacing too rapidly in deep waters. The injury was healed with HBOT treatments producing HHP.

Amir has become an indispensable partner in conceptualizing and executing our research and clinical studies for two reasons: First, he is a neurosurgeon who directly knows the look, feel, and complexity of brain structures; he has operated successfully on many patients with brain injuries and other neurological diseases. Second, he understands the brain as a medical scientist, a biologist specializing in the brain's physiology, biology, and biochemistry.

HHP can dramatically increase the volume of oxygen available to convert into what we consider the fuel of the cell—the cellular component of energy known as *adenosine triphosphate* (ATP). In brain tissue, this biochemical response, in other words the metabolism, is critical in areas being deprived of oxygen.

The volume of oxygen available for the chemical work of thinking is the principal factor limiting our capacity to put the increasing brain power of humans to work. Oxygen-rich hemoglobin and freely dissolved oxygen are transported from our beating hearts through the large carotid arteries on each side of our neck and arteries along the vertebrae in the back of our neck. If we were able to get higher volumes of oxygen into the tissues of the expanding cortex, how much would the capacity of our brain power increase?

Like a train conductor switching the engine onto different tracks to reach a specific destination, the brain carries oxygen and energy to where it is needed the most at any given moment. As we saw with those previous examples of hand movements and speaking on a phone, each time we trigger a thought or action, our brain responds in this way. It directs more oxygen through cerebral blood flow into a specific area of the cortex to execute that thought.

The mental prompt to bend and straighten the knees to perform a plié in ballet initially stimulates the supplementary motor cortex, which is responsible for planning the movement. Recalling a dinner guest's favorite dessert before they arrive activates the region of the hippocampus responsible for specific memory tasks. We call these specific cerebral destinations *areas of preference*. They are priorities framed by our biochemistry for oxygen delivery.

As the cells in our brain wear out (in medical terms, *degenerating*), these aging cells are replaced by fresh new cells (*regenerating*) all the time, just like the skin, bones, and other tissues in our bodies. We regenerate these neurons, blood vessels, and glial cells (support cells) that wear down as time passes and our bodies age chronologically. This balance between regeneration and degeneration determines the amount of active tissue in our brain.

We can see this balance between regeneration and degeneration in our skin, but it also is ongoing in other organs. For example, the full regeneration of cells in bones may take seven to ten years, but eventually all cells in our bones are replaced. In the brain, it takes at least six months for new neurons to mature.

Unfortunately, the balance shifts toward more degenerating than regenerating as we age chronologically. By the time we are in our forties, our natural physical capabilities have begun to fade as we lose some muscle tissue throughout the body (sarcopenia) and bone mass (osteoporosis).

People typically lose 1 percent of their bone mass every year after their fortieth birthday, a natural setback that can be much worse if you drink sugary or diet sodas; do little or no regular weight-bearing exercise (such as lifting weights or yoga), running, or even walking; or have an overactive thyroid. A similar decline after age forty happens in brain functions.

Brain Cells Regenerate All the Time

Some twenty years ago, most medical schools taught that neurons cannot be regenerated.[1] The existence of neural stem cells was not known. That gap in understanding our brains' physiology persuaded physicians to prescribe, and pharmaceutical companies to develop, therapies and drugs targeting specific functions of neuronal cells. Medications that target enzymes and neurotransmitters originating in neurons flowed into physicians' pharmaceutical cabinets.

Starting in the late 1990s, researchers at Rockefeller University in New York City found that the hippocampus continues to create new cells without the constraint of age or time. They showed that as hippocampus cells die, they are quickly replaced by new ones. Today, as this research has advanced, we know that damaged neurons can be regenerated and replaced by new ones, a treatment far superior to prescribing drugs targeting a specific enzyme. This is why we should aim for regeneration in treating brain injuries or disease; we should aim to repair tissue rather than relieve symptoms.

Oxygen Is a Rate-Limiting Factor for Brain Activity

We all know that any decrease in oxygen supply can threaten our cognitive functions. Take for example the impact of high altitudes. As trekkers and climbers work their way beyond 8,000 feet above sea level, they must contend with drops in barometric pressure and oxygen in the air that can affect their thinking and their judgment. For the unprepared, these stresses on physiology can impair the ability to focus as well as jostle memory, judgment, and control over emotions.

The brain's ability to perform complex tasks weakens when a pressure reading of oxygen in the arteries falls to 65 millimeters of mercury from normal readings around 100 millimeters. Things deteriorate further from there. Short-term memory becomes foggy at 55 millimeters. By the time the arterial oxygen pressure falls to 30 millimeters, fainting and loss of consciousness occurs.

Let's consider the opposite condition: Does *increasing* oxygen delivery enhance brain performance in a normal healthy person?

To answer that question, in 2017 we challenged a group of talented, fully healthy young people in their twenties to perform multiple tasks in a clinical study at the same time while breathing normal air or breathing pure oxygen at high pressure in the HBOT chamber.

The tasks included a physical movement (motor function) while attempting to solve knowledge and math problems (cognitive function). In the HBOT chamber, the test group breathed 100 percent oxygen at twice sea-level pressure (increasing their blood oxygenation about fifteen times normal levels) and another group, the control group, breathed normal air with 21 percent oxygen at normal atmospheric pressure.

The result? The test group with the higher oxygen levels scored higher in both executing physical and cognitive tasks separately and multiple tasks simultaneously. As Amir, I, and two colleagues, Dor Vadas and Leonid Kalichman, asserted in a paper for *Frontiers in Integrative Neuroscience*, "oxygen is indeed a rate-limiting factor for brain activity even in young healthy individuals."[2]

The highest concentration of neuronal stem cells is in the hippocampus, two small areas located on the medial part of the temporal lobe, at the level of our ears. The hippocampus is part of the system that controls our emotions (limbic system), short- and long-term memory, and imagination.

The high metabolic activity of the hippocampus makes it highly dependent on blood and oxygen supply. Any reduction of blood flow (ischemia) or oxygen supply (hypoxia) can shrink the hippocampus and lead to memory loss, memory disturbance, dementia, and the dreadful senile dementia of Alzheimer's disease.

Neural stem cells have the potential to generate most, if not all, different types of neurons and glial cells found in the brain. These neural stem cells multiply in numbers by dividing in two and producing either one or two kinds of offspring. In other words, neural stem cells multiply naturally by dividing in two and producing either one or two new stem cells (meaning they "self-renew") and/or one or two new daughter cells that will become a neuron or a glia cell.

Once a neuron is born, it must travel to the place in the embryonic brain where it will do its work. How does a neuron know where to go? What helps it get there? The answers to these questions enable us not only to induce proliferation of stem cells but also to target stem cells toward specific brain regions where they are most needed.

We know today that neurons in the embryo use several different methods to travel. Some migrate by following blood vessels along tubes of specific glial cells. Other neurons migrate along neuron chains, which are formed by special molecules on the surface of neurons (adhesion molecules).

The long-distance migration in one direction is guided by directional cues. Molecules serving as chemical signals usually provide these directional cues, guiding the neuron to its final location. Not all neurons succeed in their journey. In fact, most do not. It is estimated that only a third reach their destination even in a healthy embryonic brain.

Four critical supporting elements are required for a migration of newly formed neurons to succeed in reaching their destination. Three of these elements that any tissue in our body requires are: *access tracks*—arteries and veins; *energy supply*—nutritional and oxygen needed for energy generation; and *repairments*—stem cells that can replace the damaged cells. The fourth element is a system that cleans up the garbage. In other parts of the body, this is the lymphatic system. In the brain, it is the *glymphatic* system.

Glymphatic System: Cleaning up the Garbage

Not long ago, physicians believed that unlike other parts of the body, the brain had no lymphatic system (the system responsible for removing molecular waste). Well, surprise, it happens that we *do* have a biological system for removing waste in the brain. It was breakthroughs in higher resolution imaging science over the past decade that enabled scientists to uncover that biological system.

We now understand, thanks to research published in 2013 by neuroscientist Lulu Xie at the University of Rochester and thirteen colleagues, that glial cells' interactions can accelerate the rate at which waste molecules are eliminated from the brain. In their paper for *Science*, Xie and her team provided the first direct evidence of glial cells' role in eliminating waste products such as amyloid beta from extracellular connective tissue during sleep or rest.[3] (As we'll explore in chapter 10, amyloid beta is known to accumulate in brains with Alzheimer's disease.)

In the cortex, the supportive glial cells maintain the relatively stable environment (homeostasis) that our neuronal cells need to function smoothly. They are far more prevalent than neuronal cells, outnumbering neuronal cells by a factor of ten.

These glial cells have four main functions: (1) surround neurons and hold them in place; (2) supply nutrients and oxygen to neurons; (3) insulate one neuron from another; and (4) destroy any foreign microorganisms that cause disease (pathogens such as bacteria and virus) and as we like to say, clean up the garbage . . . remove dead cells (either other glia or neurons) and pathogens.

The system is active mainly during sleep. Glial cells contract and expand as muscles do, removing extra cells such as soluble proteins and small molecules (metabolites) in the brain that are no longer functioning. If we do not sleep well, the glymphatic system will not function as well as it should. Over time, poor sleeping habits degrade our mental abilities. This may be one reason why all animal species, including humans, have a biological need for sleep.

We determined through years of research that the biochemical integrity of the glymphatic system and its normal, healthy functioning is extremely important for maintaining healthy brain performance and regenerating cells to heal a damaged brain. Put another way, the glymphatic system should be one of the main therapeutical targets for physicians to evaluate for treating brain disease or injury.

Moreover, recent studies indicate that failures of the glymphatic system may be a factor in stroke, traumatic brain injury, degenerative diseases such as Alzheimer's, and other disorders of the nervous system.

New Therapies: Regeneration, Not Targeting Cell Mechanisms

Because we know that the balance between regeneration and degeneration determines our brains' performance, just as the performance of any other organ in the body is determined, we can change our therapeutic approach toward the brain just as we can with other tissues.

Instead of targeting the function of a specific cell, we understand now how to replace those damage cells with new ones through the new HBOT protocols. It is a cleaner, comprehensive process, something like replacing a flat tire with a brand-new tire rather than trying to stop the leak with an adhesive patch.

Medical scientists are developing other fascinating therapies to stimulate conditions for neuroplasticity. These therapies enable neural networks in the brain to reorganize and grow with new blood vessels, new neurons, and new connections within cells. They include creating a magnetic field in specific areas of the brain (transcranial magnetic stimulation, or TMS), manipulating genomics, injecting certain types of stem cells into the central nervous system, and creating patches that serve as a scaffold for damaged neuronal tissue to regenerate.

Our focus with clients we see at the Sagol Center for Hyperbaric Medicine and Research in Israel and our clinics in Florida and Dubai is on slowing the degenerative process as much as possible and inducing regeneration. We assess each individual's full biological profile: including their brain structure and functionality, physical fitness, metabolism, DNA, lifestyle, and diet and nutrition status.

The treatment for triggering cell regeneration and replacing damaged brain cells is framed by our new HBOT protocol in enhanced medicine. The goal is to produce the hyperoxic–hypoxic paradox; generate the hypoxic-inducible factor (HIF, or heef); and produce the surge of stem cells, mitochondria number and function, and angiogenesis (creation of new blood vessels).

In the rest of Part II, we will explore six common types of brain injuries. For each of these, we will sketch the cascade of events that can damage brain tissue (pathophysiology), describe treatments currently available, and explain the newly developed therapies.

Key Takeaways

1. The brain is a tissue. As in any other tissue in our body, cells in our brain are being replaced by new ones all along our lifespan. Net brain performance at any stage of life is the balance between degenerating and regenerating these cells.

2. The volume of oxygen available for the chemical work of thinking is the principal factor that limits our capacity to put the increasing brain power of humans to work.

3. The human cortex continues to expand with each new generation, leading to ever-higher cognitive potential. There has been a *threefold* increase in human brain size in a mere 2.5 million years.

CHAPTER 5

Stroke

The day I finished my four-year residency in internal medicine, I started a new residency in nephrology that would require another three years of training. Malignant hypertension was one kidney disease that particularly interested me. I had my sights set on becoming an expert.

An episode of malignant hypertension is a medical emergency that can trigger cell death in any part of the body—the brain, the heart, the kidney, and more. It most often afflicts people with high blood pressure, but it can happen to other people as well. It is more common in young adults, especially among Black people.

Kidneys are such important organs in orchestrating the blood pressure, electrolytes, and biochemistry for how well the body functions or does not function. Nephrology is a specialty in how kidneys function, renal-related disease, electrolyte balance, fluid-volume balance, and blood pressure; each is a dynamic element of homeostasis.

Homeostasis is the self-regulating process by which biological systems tend to maintain stability while adjusting to conditions that are optimal for survival. If homeostasis is successful, life continues; if unsuccessful, disaster or death ensues. Accordingly, nephrologists are expected to acquire an encyclopedic understanding of human physiology, one of the main reasons I was drawn to it. When the kidney stops functioning, nephrologists take full control to preserve the human homeostasis.

To understand the exact biological cascade that the abrupt increase in blood pressure initiates and then culminates in cell death, I needed to simulate in the laboratory this abrupt increase at the cellular level. I designed a chamber in which I could expose different cells to an increase in pressure, but I needed someone to help me build it. Luckily, that help was just down the hall.

Physicians knew at the time that breathing pure oxygen at above-normal pressure—hyperbaric oxygen—successfully healed visible wounds caused by insufficient blood flow and oxygen supply, such as diabetic ulcers in legs.

A technical team in my hospital that was helping physicians treat diabetic patients with foot ulcers and leg wounds agreed to build the smaller laboratory version for my experiments with kidneys and malignant hypertension.

This smaller chamber immediately became a convenient place for me to simulate the impact of sudden surges in blood pressure on those cells. Moreover, as a diver myself, active in Israel's medical society for diving, I was curious about the physiology applications of a hyper-pressurized environment.

It wasn't long before I learned that the hospital's hyperbaric unit was not operating at its best with respect to logistics and service. One day the hospital manager approached me and said, "Shai, you're having success with the research unit you have established. Why don't you take over the hyperbaric unit? Maybe we could do better."

I immediately thought to myself, *No way!* I was practically living at the hospital at the time, juggling duties as a resident physician, seeing patients, and mentoring colleagues as activity in my kidney research unit was beginning to surge. I also was the medical director of a small company that was bringing to market a promising new technology for patients who need mechanical ventilation in intensive care units (ICUs), post-operative recovery, and other wards.[1]

"I have plenty on my table already," I told the manager. "I can't do that." But he continued pressing me.

"Change your mind. Take on the hyperbarics unit."

I kept turning him down. After a month of this, he told me flatly, "Shai, the unit is not successful. I'm losing money. I cannot hold it open anymore, so I will close it."

"You can't do that!" I protested. I was exasperated. "Where will these people with the diabetic wounds go for treatment? There aren't any other hospitals around here that have a hyperbaric facility."

"I don't know," he said. "But I am closing that unit."

Along my journey in life, I had come to believe by then that if you have the opportunity to do something good and you're not doing it, it's just as if you are doing something bad. If you are not exploring the opportunity to do something good, the universe will hit you. But if you *are* doing something good, somehow things will go along okay. New doors will open for you. It's better to do good.

"Okay," I said to the manager, muttering an expletive. "Leave it open. I will be responsible for the hyperbaric unit. I can make something out of it."

It was when I began taking more interest in the hyperbarics operations, the equipment, staff, and patients that I first noticed the patient I describe at the beginning of chapter 1. She'd had a stroke years earlier and now was out of her wheelchair, walking around the hospital's small hyperbaric chamber for diabetics.

Professional ethics required that I design at least one study with stroke patients and hyperbarics after I observed the same thing: two other stroke patients walking in the chamber. So, I did. *Once I finished,* I reassured myself, *I'll be clear with the universe and free to resume my research in kidney disease.*

I felt certain the study would prove there was *no connection* between hyperbarics treatments for post-stroke recoveries I'd witnessed. In medical science terms, I anticipated it would demonstrate that it is impossible through hyperbaric oxygen therapy to induce neuroplasticity; meaning, to regenerate and rearrange patterns in how neurons communicate and to restore lost brain functions at the late chronic stage.

A Study We Anticipated Would Fail

In the early months, it was extremely difficult to persuade people who had suffered a stroke to participate. We talked with neurologists and physical therapists who worked with these patients, hoping they'd send us recruits. We needed patients at least six months past their stroke. Why six months? Spontaneous natural recovery of some weakened capacities can happen up to three months. After six months, there was little chance any participant in our study could experience a significant spontaneous recovery. That type of change could muddy our conclusions of whether HBOT did or did not help stroke patients. We then would need a smaller study cohort, or sample size, to prove the point.

Recruiting was hard because neurologists and rehabilitation therapists were skeptical of the study's premise: that a surge of oxygen and energy delivered through HBOT can stimulate growth of neurons, repair damaged ones, and restore brain and motor functions lost after a stroke.

Of course, at that point, *I was skeptical, too*—and said so.

I went on to stress my ethical obligation to explore the physiology behind the recoveries I had observed in those three diabetic patients. Were they related to HBOT or not? Over time, as word of the overwhelmingly positive results from the first patients to finish treatment spread among neurologists and rehabilitation groups, more stroke patients volunteered to be included in the study. We had to turn some away.

The study encompassed seventy-four patients. Each had suffered a stroke between six months and three years prior. To simplify things, we recruited patients with some type of motor problem that we could visually assess. They would be unable to move a hand, leg, or finger or take care of routine daily living tasks such as cooking, eating, and toileting.

The group tapped for the HBOT had forty ninety-minute sessions, five days a week over two months to generate the hyperoxic–hypoxic paradox (HHP). The control continued with their standard rehabilitation. As we wrote in our January 2013 journal article, patients in the treatment group had "statistically significant improvements" from their debilitating impacts after stroke.[2] They now could better raise a hand or lift an arm or leg. There was no significant improvement in the control group. Later, after the study finished, we offered the same complete HBOT protocol for patients in the control group. Their results matched those of the initial treatment group. We were thrilled.

I knew my decade-long dreams for research breakthroughs in kidney disease and high blood pressure were being derailed. Experimenting with fluctuations of elevated pressure and oxygen concentration in the hyperbaric chamber led me to an entirely new direction: adapting HBOT to induce HHP, hypoxia-inducible factor (HIF), and the regeneration of damaged brain tissue.

Recovery through HBOT a Year after Stroke

A sixty-one-year-old woman who entered the treatment group had suffered an ischemic stroke a year earlier. She could not lift her left hand at all (against gravity) and could only lift her left leg for a few seconds. She needed help bathing, dressing, and climbing stairs and could not do any housework. Her face was partially paralyzed, and she had lost some ability to see and hear clearly.

After receiving the HBOT protocol—her biochemistry stimulated through HHP and HIF—she was able to lift her hand and leg comfortably and move her fingers. She regained much of her pre-stroke acuity in vision and hearing. The net effect on her daily activities was a return to independence. She could bathe and dress herself and do her own grocery shopping and cooking.

The images in Figure 5-1 show how oxygen flows to areas of her brain weakened from the stroke improved during the hyperbarics treatments.

The Disability, Symptoms, and Science of Stroke

Strokes can be disabling in many ways, with varying degrees of severity. Difficulty with speech or reading, loss of vision, loss of hand, fingers, arm, or leg movement on one side of the body, and diminished memory and other cognitive functions are common.

Medical evaluations for assessing a stroke's severity cover all these functions: bathing, dressing, grooming, oral care, toileting, walking, climbing stairs, eating, shopping, cooking, managing medications, using a phone, housework, doing laundry, driving, and managing finances.

Patients become despondent often when the effects of a stroke make it impossible for them to handle simple daily habits such as bathing, dressing, and using the toilet. They lose independence.

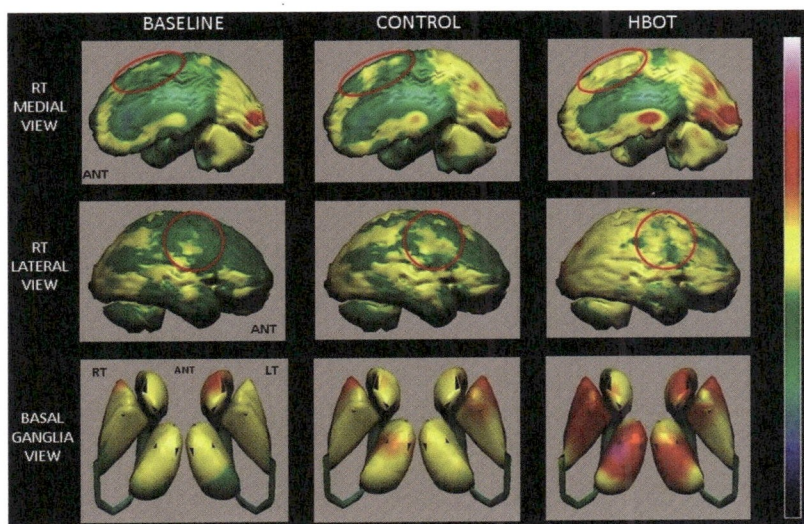

Figure 5-1: The baseline and control images (top two rows: upper left and center, respectively) show with red circles in green areas where restricted blood flows had limited her hand and leg movement before the treatments. The HBOT images (top two rows, upper right) indicate how in widening yellow areas blood flows were restored after the treatments.

Every forty seconds, someone in the United States suffers a stroke, what some medical professionals now refer to as a "brain attack." That stunning frequency adds up to nearly 800,000 cases per year, according to the Centers for Disease Control and Prevention.[3] Every three and a half minutes, someone dies from a stroke.[4]

There are two types of strokes. One is ischemic, a condition in which blood clots or some other blockage (occlusion) in an artery restricts or prevents oxygen flows in some area of the brain and disrupts the functions, such as memory or motor movement, controlled in that area. Ischemic stroke is by far the more common type, totaling about 87 percent of all strokes in the United States. The other type is hemorrhagic, a rupture somewhere in the wall of an artery that causes blood to leak into adjacent areas of the brain.

Leaking Blood, Rising Pressure in a Closed Box

For an ischemic stroke, we want to remove the blockage, which most often is a blood clot, as soon as possible. We do this either with drugs to break up the clot (thrombolytic therapy), or by inserting a tiny tube into the arteries, maneuvering the tube to the precise location of the blockage, and removing the clot. The major danger from brain hemorrhage arises as leaking blood seeps into places it does not belong.

This pressure building inside the skull—a closed box with the brain inside—can damage neurons and other tissue. Blood flows through the arteries according to a pressure gradient, meaning from areas of high pressure toward lower pressure. When a hemorrhage causes pressure in the closed box to increase, the gradient decreases and the blood and oxygen supply falls. Mental or motor functions controlled in that section of the brain can break down.

How can we reduce rising pressure caused by blood leaking from the ruptured vein or artery? One method is opening a section of the skull by removing part of the scalp. A second is drilling a hole in the skull. Another is inserting a stent into a leaking artery and inflating its tiny balloon to fit the artery wall and prevent blood from leaking.

After a stroke occurs, physicians counsel patients to limit factors that may have caused that stroke and prevent another one. Primary reasons for stroke include high blood pressure, high cholesterol, obesity and diabetes, and smoking. For stroke patients, physical therapy, fitness training, and cognitive training with mental exercises are vital elements that we need to "teach" healthy tissues in the brain to take on diminished functions of damaged tissues.

One of the most important results of our first HBOT study for stroke patients was that it made clear what HBOT in enhanced medicine *cannot* do. HBOT cannot revive dead tissue in the brain; dead tissue is replaced with cerebral spinal fluid, leaving no space for angiogenesis and the restorative benefits that could be delivered by migration of higher levels of stem cells.

The analogy we use with clients to describe this limitation is that triggering HHP can be like putting a cast on your broken leg. A cast will help heal the broken leg. But if you have had to have an amputation, and the full leg is no longer there, a cast won't help heal the leg. It's the same with dead tissue in the brain. HHP cannot help heal dead tissue in the brain. Our natural biochemistry, in effect, has "amputated" that dead tissue. That dead tissue cannot function.

This study showed us for the first time that physicians need to approach the brain as a tissue as they would with any other tissue. We need to evaluate wounds in the brain just as we do for wounds in any other part of the body. Any clinical improvement that resolves a dysfunction in some tissue happens because its metabolism, the life-sustaining chemical reactions in that tissue, has been restored. If the tissue is damaged, we can recover it. If the tissue is dead, it's lost.

Stroke Warning Signs and Quick Actions

A handful of symptoms are often signals about the onset of a stroke. Rapid action to alert emergency responders with a call to 9-1-1 can save lives and enable medical professionals to reverse stroke symptoms safely if treatment is applied within three hours after the symptoms are recognized and diagnosed.

The CDC lists these five warning signs of stroke in men and women:

1. Sudden numbness or weakness in the face, arm, or leg, especially on one side of the body
2. Sudden confusion, trouble speaking, or difficulty understanding speech

3. Sudden trouble seeing in one or both eyes
4. Sudden trouble walking, dizziness, loss of balance, or lack of coordination
5. Sudden severe headache with no known cause

If you think you or someone near you may be having a stroke, the CDC urges taking these actions as quickly as possible. To underscore the critical value of rapid diagnosis and treatment, the steps by CDC are bundled under the acronym FAST.

- **F—Face:** Ask the person to smile. Does one side of the face droop?
- **A—Arms:** Ask the person to raise both arms. Does one arm drift downward?
- **S—Speech:** Ask the person to repeat a simple phrase. Is the speech slurred or strange?
- **T—Time:** If you see any of these signs, call 9-1-1 right away.

A Breakthrough in Visualizing Brain Damage

A brilliant physics professor in Tel Aviv, Eshel Ben-Jacob, was in many ways the father of the amazing visualization capabilities we have in brain imaging today. We can display for any patient in our clinics detailed sections of tissue (such as functional magnetic resonant imaging, or fMRI) or three-dimensional images of tissues (single-photon emission computer tomography, or SPECT).

Eshel had become fascinated with the research and treatments we were developing in 2012 for stroke patients and asked me how he could help. I replied, "You know, we need some way to demonstrate that the brain is a tissue, too."

He answered, "That's on me. I'll use my expertise in physics. I will figure it out."

And he did. He created algorithms that through their coding could interpret hard data and translate insights from that data visually in colors that made brain injury simpler for physicians to see and explain to patients. This advance gave us the technology to demonstrate and illustrate visually the brain's anatomy and metabolic functions. I'll have more to say about Prof. Ben-Jacob and our early collaborations shortly.

How HBOT Can Improve the Effects of Stroke

As we've seen, a stroke can often leave the patient with two degrees of brain injuries. The most severe is necrosis, or fully dead tissue, which as we've established cannot be recovered even in enhanced medicine with HBOT. However, in some areas the injury may be less severe and a chronic penumbra, or "stunned" brain tissue, is formed.

Cells in these stunned areas do have the minimal amount of energy necessary to survive, but they cannot generate enough energy required for normal function in the injured area of the brain. In medical terms, those cells have metabolic dysfunction. The stunned area usually surrounds the initial core of the necrotic tissue. It happens that, unlike what we thought in the past, this stagnated state can persist for years, hence the adjective *chronic*.

By improving oxygenation as HBOT treatments generate the hyperoxic–hypoxic paradox within these "border zones" of necrotic tissue, we can rejuvenate neurons previously regarded as nonfunctional. For stroke patients in particular, when selected appropriately, HBOT has been proven to induce neuroplasticity—the brain's ability to reorganize the synaptic connections of neurons—even years after the acute stroke. With brain imaging, we can observe this improvement during three months of HBOT treatments as more oxygen and stem cells reach the areas with metabolic dysfunction.

The brain images in Figure 5-2[5] show the progress of a seventy-two-year-old man with muscle weakness or partial paralysis on the right side of his body (right hemiparesis) due to an ischemic stroke he suffered thirty-four months prior to starting our HBOT protocol.

The baseline examination showed his lack of strength to hold his right leg and hand against gravity. Also, he could say single words but not complete sentences (moderate aphasia). After treatment he had significant improvement in the motor function of both his hand and leg as well as more strength to hold them both against gravity. He had laudable improvement in his fine motor skills and his language communication was much better as well; he regained the ability to complete sentences.

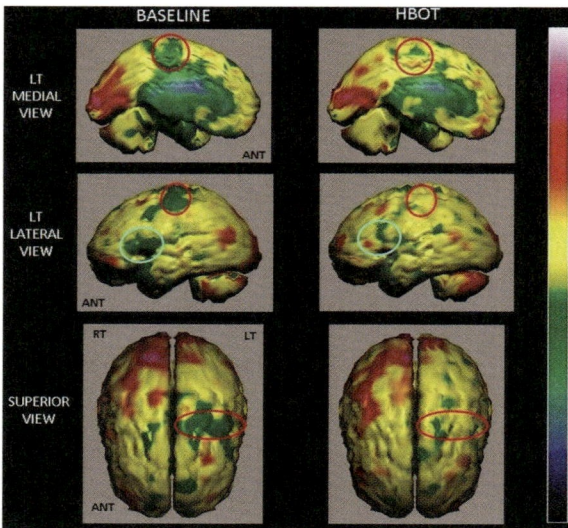

Figure 5-2

Broadly speaking, brain imaging at different phases of HHP treatments will demonstrate improved metabolism in stroke patients as it occurs in areas of the brain that control both motor and speech functions and that correlate with the patient's recovering physical capabilities.

Although the main focus in post-stroke patients is usually on motor function, up to 50 percent of stroke survivors suffer from cognitive deficits. In another study, we examined the cognitive domains of stroke survivors using an objective computerized assessment battery.

This study demonstrated that our HBOT protocol can significantly improve the cognitive functions of post-stroke patients. Moreover, the full spectrum of cognitive activity—memory, executive function, attention, information processing, and speed—significantly increased regardless of the stroke origin, type, or location.

These studies' results illustrate the benefits of HHP and HIF and transform our preconceived notions of the type of cognitive improvements that are possible for patients in the chronic late stage following stroke. Moreover, these findings reinforced the previous conclusion that the main factor for cognitive improvement was patients' selection based on metabolic dysfunction on brain imaging.

Paired with a Master

As word spread of our HBOT clinical study's unanticipated positive results in reversing neurological damage from stroke, an inspiring, highly successful industrialist came to meet with me, intrigued. He told me he was considering a major donation, a gift that would give me resources to dramatically accelerate this work into a disciplined new path of brain injury research.

I explained to him the study findings, the biochemical responses to HBOT that can repair some of the stroke damage and the implications for HHP as a medical breakthrough potentially for treating many types of neurological brain injuries. These ideas were novel, unexamined by medical peers. The next time we met, he brought with him one of Israel's preeminent physicists, someone to probe, understand, and assess my scientific thinking. Were these ideas logical? Was the potential for breakthroughs significant?

That physicist was Prof. Eshel Ben-Jacob. In my mind, as we chatted for the first time, it was clear that he was the superstar, and I was the amateur. After we spoke for several hours, he said, "Shai, I want to spend more time with you. I want to be your shadow for a couple of days. Just to watch what you do." He was with me as I met and counseled patients, shared research ideas with my team, and pored through new research that might help advance my thinking.

At the end of that week, as we sat alone together, he said quietly, "Shai, I want to join you and have impact on human health and improving physiological performance. These are the truly important matters of life. We have a huge opportunity here to make a difference in the lives of millions of people around the world. I want to be part of this journey. I will do whatever is needed."

I was in shock. This man was a brilliant mathematician and physicist, one of the top scientists in our society. *He was willing to dedicate his energy and scientific insights to our HBOT research?*

It was a huge honor when Eshel emphatically endorsed the science behind our research. The intrigued industrialist, Sami Sagol, quickly became a transitional force, providing the mental support, the scale-up thinking, and the foundational funding that has helped make possible our progressing HHP research for the past ten years. Our work together—a mission shared by the three of us—was cut short far too soon. Eshel, one of the

authors for the article describing the seminal stroke patient study, suc-
cumbed to cancer a few years later.

With Brain Imaging, Seeing Is Believing

These images make a stronger impact than any statistics we might
have. We could show a client or patient where something in the brain
was amiss, where tissue was not fully dead, and explain how HBOT
and other treatments would help resolve a metabolic dysfunction from
that brain injury.

Before this breakthrough, physicians had to rely on technicians
to collect and interpret data from a standard MRI of anything in
the brain. Texts of those interpretations often were difficult to
understand. This made diagnosis and treatment challenging. On
the other hand, when physicians assessed a leg wound, they could
form an initial diagnosis immediately. If tissue was black, it was
necrotic—it was dead. "Intermittent" or vaguely green areas with
reduced oxygen supply were damaged but still had a chance of
recovery.

Newer imaging technology, MRI with DTI (magnetic resonance imaging and diffusion tensor tractography) enables us to see
and assess the integrity of nerve fibers, the microstructure of the
brain. The techniques illuminate pathways as multicolored fibers.
In perfusion MRI, we can use whatever array of colors we choose
to illustrate varying blood flows and oxygen delivery in different
areas of the brain. The perfusion MRI correlates with metabolic
activity, while the MRI-DTI correlates with the microstructure of
nerve fibers.

By simplifying functional imaging of the brain, these technologies
made it possible to demonstrate that the brain is a tissue and can be
treated as a tissue. Even if you are not a professional, you can see the

condition inside the brain just as if you were looking at a wound on the body.

Today in medicine, advanced brain imaging continues to confirm our approach: the four basic things we need to repair and heal a visible wound on the body are the same basic things we need to heal wounds inside our head.

1. We need energy.
2. We need a trigger to start our biological repair cascade.
3. We need stem cells.
4. We need new blood vessels (angiogenesis).

This first HBOT clinical study with stroke patients emerged from that extreme case—witnessing those unexpected moments of patients treated with HBOT for diabetic leg wounds regaining the ability lost from stroke to walk and move their hands and legs again. Because we pursued the science behind it, this study became the seminal investigation affirming that the brain is a tissue.

As we summarized on the concluding page of our scientific paper, "In this study we provide, for the first time, convincing results demonstrating that HBOT can induce significant neurological improvement in post-stroke patients. The neurological improvements in a chronic late stage demonstrate that neuroplasticity can be operative and activated by HBOT even long after acute brain insult. Thus, the findings have important implications that can be of general relevance and interest in neurobiology. Although this study focused on stroke patients, the findings bear promise that HBOT may serve as a valuable therapeutic practice in other neurological disorders exhibiting discrepancy between the anatomical and functional evaluation of the brain."[6]

And indeed, it has.

I could hardly have been more wrong about the anticipated outcome—and the importance—of that study with stroke patients. The results, published in 2013, opened new pathways for me and many others to examine the potential of these treatments for healing an array of brain injuries. What we learned suggested a vastly higher significance for HBOT, HHP, and HIF in medicine beyond treating stroke. That's really the story of the rest of this book.

As we will see in the next chapters of Part II, the promise of our HBOT protocol as a valuable therapeutic practice for other neurological disorders continues to be demonstrated.

Key Takeaways

1. Our first HBOT study for post-stroke patients, completed in 2010, demonstrated that neuroplasticity can be activated and operative even long after a stroke event.
2. Physicians need to approach the brain as a tissue as they would with any other tissue. We need to evaluate wounds in the brain just as we do for wounds in any other part of the body.
3. Brain imaging for different patients demonstrated that the positive effects induced by HBOT and HHP occurred in the injured, not fully necrotic (dead) brain regions.
4. New imaging techniques make it possible for us to characterize wounds in the brain in ways similar to how we characterize wounds in other parts of our body.

CHAPTER 6

Concussion

E xcited as we were by the stroke study's results confirming HBOT's healing potential, we were uncertain about where to focus our research next.

The study gave us insight into the type of brain wounds that might benefit most from HHP and HIF. Our biggest breakthrough was confirming that brain regions with reduced oxygen supply and diminished metabolism can recover much or all their lost potency.

They retain a biological infrastructure on which stem cells can migrate and differentiate into the missing tissue and new blood vessels can grow. We were able to demonstrate those depleted areas by combining brain metabolic imaging (SPECT) with anatomical imaging such as standard magnetic resonance imaging (MRI) or computerized tomography (CT).

By 2010, we had decided to follow up the stroke study with a similar examination of how our HBOT protocol might benefit patients with another neurological injury, post-concussion syndrome, or PCS.

People in our medical network in Israel who had learned about stroke patients' recoveries in the HBOT test group and knew of others with PCS who recovered after HBOT treatment urged us to assemble a similar random-control study for PCS patients.

The medically sound, positive results for patients in the trial group and their implications for continuing our HBOT research on other neurological diseases are the story of this chapter.

Examining a Disturbing Persistence: Post-Concussion Syndrome

In most cases, the headaches, dizziness, cognitive decline, mental fatigue, vertigo, mood changes, and other disorienting impacts after a concussion fade away after a week or two. We classify these as mild traumatic brain injuries, or mTBI. Life returns to normal for about four of every five people who experience mild-to-moderate traumatic brain injury or jolt to the head. But what about the rest who make up roughly 25 percent of the people impacted by concussion injuries? For them, the disorienting effects of PCS can extend for months, years, or even become permanent for the rest of their lives.

The deteriorating quality of life for concussion patients who do not recover becomes so significant that they can become extremely frustrated. They become despondent if they are unable to return to satisfying work, retain their normal cognitive functions, or maintain friendships and supporting social networks. Meanwhile, their families can be staggered by the physical, financial, and emotional shockwaves that PCS can trigger.

PCS symptoms continue to be misdiagnosed too frequently as emotional or psychological problems. We in the medical profession had missed the biological problem because our way of looking at the brain was too limited. The magnitude of biological damage could not be seen with standard brain imaging tools of CT or MRI, so many physicians routinely and erroneously insisted to a patient that they did not have a "real" biological brain injury; they "only" had an emotional problem. That would increase a patient's frustration even more.

Traumatic brain injury (TBI) has become a major public health concern globally for both civilian and military populations, with at least ten million new head injuries occurring annually. It is a leading cause of death and disability in the United States, with an estimated average of 1.4 million cases per year; of these, 50,000 will not survive a severe TBI, 235,000 will be hospitalized, and the remaining 1.1 million will be treated and discharged from emergency departments.[1] Less severe but still dangerous, concussions are more prevalent, typically stemming from motor vehicle accidents (50 percent), falls (38 percent), sports injuries, and violence, including attempted suicide.

There are no accurate statistics on mild TBI because most people with this concussion injury don't go to a hospital, and 25 percent of those who do are never reevaluated beyond the time of the injury.[2] According to the Centers for Disease Control and Prevention, more than five million Americans, or about 2 percent of the population, are living with long-term disabilities resulting from TBI.[3]

Sports-Related Injuries

Concussions suffered during sports and recreation activities each year amount to between 1.7 and 3 million cases; football drills and competitions beginning in elementary school and up through professional teams contribute 300,000 of those.[4,5]

News accounts since 2007 have chronicled sobering declines in the personal lives of former professional football players in the United States who struggled with escalating mood disorders, paranoia, memory loss, and an array of erratic behaviors, such as explosive rages.

Brain analyses after some of their deaths showed evidence of chronic traumatic encephalopathy, or CTE, a progressive degenerative disease linked to repetitive blows to the head over many years that in some cases may have led to former players' suicides.[6]

Blast Injuries in Military Settings

Soldiers also are highly vulnerable to concussions and complex neurological impacts from blast injuries. Blast waves release light, sound, heat, and electromagnetic energy that, combined with effects of the ultrasound pressure wave, can damage the central nervous system. Abrupt pressure changes inflicted on the brain can cause bubbles to form in extracellular fluids of the brain. These bubbles can damage the brain's surface and produce a shock wave through brain matter, as well as impair capillaries, lodge in blood vessels, and reduce blood flows. Each of the latter three can starve tissue of oxygen.

The Pentagon puts the number of military service members diagnosed with TBI between 2000 and 2019 at more than 400,000. U.S. military officials regard TBI as the signature injury of the Afghanistan and Iraq military conflicts; with 28 percent of soldiers evacuated diagnosed. Risks in combat zones had exposed many—especially on foot patrols—to stunning explosions, often from remote-controlled devices that propel shock waves of highly compressed air. Helmets offered some protection, but not much. Three-fourths of soldiers who sustained any type of TBI were wearing helmets when they suffered these injuries.

Most diagnoses, which are reported overwhelmingly by the U.S. Army in contrast to other branches, came directly from active soldiers or veterans who sought medical help for hearing problems or headaches. Psychological setbacks often followed, typically from depression and post-traumatic stress disorder (PTSD), but episodes of anxiety and troubles with sleep, focus, and clear thinking are also common.*

The Science of Concussion

What happens to the normal physiology inside the head when you have a concussion?

In addition to fluids, the brain has two major layers of tissue: the cortex, the outside layer, and the medulla, the inner layer. The cortex is composed mainly of the cells that we refer to commonly as *gray matter*, while the medulla is composed mostly of exons, the connecting fiber transferring the signal from one neuronal cell to another.

Football helmets repeatedly colliding, foreheads stunned in a car accident, or, as we saw with Dylan Hartley in chapter 2, head-on-head rugby clashes, a sudden blast near soldiers on foot patrol, or other serious blows to the head resulting in concussion all trigger Newton's second law of physics. This is the basic equation of motion: a force acting on a body is equal to the mass of the body multiplied by the acceleration of the body; or, force is equal to mass times acceleration (F = ma). Millions of small blood vessels and long connecting fibers (axons) are stressed by the friction. Many may rupture. The gray matter–white matter junctions in the frontal and temporal (side) lobes are the most vulnerable sites.

---

* The Pentagon's soaring medical bill to care for soldiers with TBIs followed the surge in battlefield incidents as the total cost of care rose to approximately $646 million in 2010. Lifetime costs for treating one patient with TBI can range from $85,000 to more than $3 million. The financial burden of TBI on individuals, families, national economies, and health systems has been estimated at $56 billion per year.

Imaging Captures
Before–After Impact of HBOT

In this illustration, we can see brain images of a fifty-one-year-old woman who suffered a concussion (mild traumatic brain injury, or mTBI) in a fall from a bus. The incident happened two years before her HBOT treatment.

Images in the baseline row show her concussion injuries in green and yellow colors depicting areas deprived or depleted of oxygen. The post-HBOT images in the bottom row show in red how HBOT induced a broad recovery in most of those injured areas.

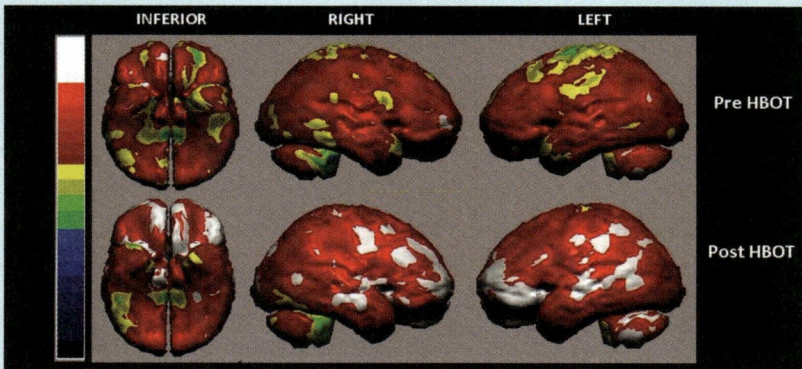

Figure 6-1

Oxygen supplies fall where this happens as blood flows decline (hypoxia). Any tissues starved of oxygen cannot function normally as the volume of available energy plummets as mitochondria fail. However, in 80 to 90 percent of concussions, blood vessel damage is slight, the tissue can recover, and the initial symptoms such as fatigue and memory loss fade within a week or two. Most people recover.

But when concussion friction severs too many small blood vessels, areas impacted by the diminished oxygen supplies become a bottleneck that prevents or substantially slows healing. Symptoms related to the damage to these biochemical pathways and brain structures may continue for weeks or months in 10 to 20 percent of the cases. Among those patients, 25 to 33 percent develop a more permanent brain injury.

Many patients will struggle for years or even the rest of their lives with neuropsychiatric disorders such as depression, anxiety, memory and attention difficulties, and mood and impulse troubles. These setbacks complicate their ability to manage daily functions on their own such as eating, bathing, and dressing. As we just noted, the diagnosis of chronic traumatic encephalopathy, or CTE, closely identified with former football players is a progressive degenerative syndrome.

What is unfolding is permanent brain injury, an unfortunate cascade of biochemical tragedy. Areas starved for oxygen after a concussion suffer cell death or chronic inflammation. There is a breakdown in energy production from disrupted mitochondria activity and a decline of the brain's biochemical activity. These accumulating malfunctions cause the vitality of synapses and neurons to fade along with molecular communications between neurons.

Investigating HBOT and Post-Concussion Syndrome

Diagnosing PCS is not easy. For one thing, as mentioned, standard brain scans from CT and MRI will not show any significant damage from mTBI. Moreover, scientifically measuring whether someone's cognitive ability declined or whether any mood patterns, such as depression or anxiety, existed before the concussion or became more pronounced due to damage in the frontal lobe is rarely possible.

We required all patients screened for the HBOT-PCS study to have metabolic imaging by a specific SPECT scan of their brains, an advancing technology that was well established by 2008. These methods, such as perfusion MRI, monitoring radioactive tracers in positron emission tomography (PET), or SPECT scans enable us to see brain regions with metabolic dysfunctions in an objective manner. Both measure brain activity by identifying changes associated with blood flows to tissues.

We couldn't rely on someone's perception that a concussion was causing them mental or physical problems. We needed to *see* the metabolic dysfunction—the brain tissue wounds—with advanced SPECT images that can detect altered or blocked blood flows. The goal was to objectively evaluate whether there is damage in the brain. Some patients cried tears of joy when I showed them images confirming concussion brain damage.

They were profoundly excited, relieved to know they had not been imagining the post-concussion mental and physical struggles that were pulling them down. While screening patients to be certain they had a metabolic dysfunction in some area of the brain, we also needed to be confident they had no unresolved issues with their medical insurance provider related to compensation for the incident that caused the brain injury. Any claim had to have been settled.

Our first clinical study on the use of HBOT for healing concussion damage was initiated in 2010. The results: more than fifty participants with PCS showed significant improvement in their speed in processing information as well as their attention (focus), memory, and executive functions.

As usual in a randomized study, we separated the participants initially into two groups, one receiving treatment and one in a control group. To gauge each participant's response, a computerized neurocognitive evaluation gave us first a baseline and then progressive comparisons of their thinking and reasoning capabilities. Then, too, responses to a questionnaire assessed their current quality of life, and we executed brain imaging with SPECT scans.

I thought results for both groups were amazing. I always challenge my students to ask themselves, *When do I know that some treatment I've studied is working?* They usually answer with a technical term that measures the statistical probability that a different hypothesis could explain the results—the p value. The right answer, I tell them, is, "You know something is working when there is no need for statistical analysis, even though we still do it. When somebody you've treated tells you, 'I am fully recovered,' then it is clear."

When a patient tells you they are fully recovered, this is the greatest reward you can experience as a physician. Most participants in the PCS clinical study indeed fully recovered. As expected, there was no significant improvement for participants in the control group during the control period.

After these participants completed their final evaluation for the two-month study, we allowed all of them to receive the same full HBOT protocol we had given to the treatment group. They also improved.

As we wrote in the paper describing the study, "It seems reasonable to let patients benefit from HBOT now rather than wait until future studies are completed."[7] That study was repeated later in the United States, with similar positive results for participants,[8] and additional data was accumulated by us and by others across the globe.

A Horrific Train Disaster and Five Years of Concussion Misdiagnosis

One participant in the post-concussion study had to be coaxed into it.

Shir Daphna-Tekoah was riding on a passenger train in 2005 when the train rammed into a forty-ton coal truck. Eight people died and 200 were injured in one of Israel's worst train disasters. The carriage she was seated in flipped twice. She was propelled outside into a field of sunflowers. Shir had several physical injuries—an injured leg, headaches, backaches—and a concussion from a brain injury that would not be correctly diagnosed until we met five years later.

During those years, she felt certain that all the physicians and psychiatrists she consulted were wrong. They had diagnosed her extreme fatigue, memory loss, unrelenting physical pain, and alarmingly failing cognitive abilities as PTSD symptoms. These professionals prescribed multiple medications and regular physical therapy such as swimming in hot water.

"For five years, I had been walking on the path of people losing their minds," she says, a subject she understood in great depth. Shir had already completed a master's degree in psychoanalysis at Oxford University and had just finished her first year of studies for a PhD in childhood sexual trauma at the time of the train accident.

"Nothing in the health system had given me any hope. My body was painful and weak. I was full of medicines. After the rehabilitation, speech therapy, physical therapy, and more, I was not seeing any improvement. My mind was failing. My photographic memory was gone. I couldn't recall any English words. In my lectures, I forgot terms even in Hebrew."

A lawyer friend had recently assessed her ailments as related to concussion, not PTSD, and after a professional colleague learned about our promising HBOT stroke study, she called our clinic. A member of our team in the clinic walked her through our HBOT procedures and encouraged her to volunteer for a new study we were planning on the effects of HBOT on PCS.

But she was wary. "I didn't want to go into any hyperbaric treatments, just the screening to see if I indeed had had a concussion," she recalls. "My husband is a PhD microbiologist. He was concerned that hyperbarics treatments generate free radicals."[†]

---

† Free radicals are atom pairs, electrons that might be associated with cell damage in a variety of diseases.

I assured Shir there was no risk of free-radical damage with our new HBOT protocol and noted that a free SPECT brain scan was part of the screening regimen for all participants. She eventually agreed to be one of the participants. "Everyone had been saying I had post-traumatic stress disorder, but I knew this was not true. I am a researcher of trauma. I had no fear when riding trains. If I had PTSD from the train disaster, how could I ride on trains?"

As we reviewed the SPECT images of her brain trauma together, I pointed to the ischemic areas lacking oxygen. These images were inspiring to me in one sense, stunning in another. I was amazed she had been able to struggle with and complete her PhD, a dissertation on psychiatric disorders related to childhood sexual abuse, in the same years she confronted such a serious brain injury. I told her, "You are a phenomenon. How were you able to do this?" She began to cry.

"I felt that after so many years, now someone understood, someone who knows what he is doing," she said later, recalling the moment. "I thought, *Now I can breathe. I know the problem.*" After her first week of sessions in the hyperbaric chamber, she said, "My brain felt like dust had cleared after a fresh rain. Everything became bright. After a month of treatment, I felt less weak."

Shir completed what in that 2010 clinical study was a two-month, forty-session HBOT treatment with substantial recovery.[‡] "I came for help with my brain and gained back my body and control of my life again." Control is an understatement. She reclaimed her acclaimed academic and lecturing skills on psychological trauma and childhood sexual abuse so thoroughly that she is now a professor and dean of the faculty of social work at Israel's Ashkelon Academic College.

[‡] "Report to Congress on Mild Traumatic Brain Injury in the United States: Steps to Prevent a Serious Public Health Problem," National Center for Injury Prevention and Control, 2003.

Healing people such as Shir in this way not only affects their own life, it also allows them to honor their own purpose to help others in their lifetime.

As we will see in the next chapter, Shir urged us after finishing the post-concussion syndrome study to examine HBOT's effects on another much misunderstood and misdiagnosed brain injury—fibromyalgia. She had suffered a multitude of fibromyalgia pains following the train disaster *until* the HBOT post-concussion treatments unexpectedly quieted them during and after the 2010 clinical study.

HBOT Is Also Effective for Post-Concussion Symptoms in Children

Mild traumatic brain injuries (mTBIs) affect more than 10 percent of children under the age of sixteen. Bicycle and vehicle accidents, falls as well as sports injuries and blunt force trauma are principal causes. Most recover completely within a few weeks, but as many as 25 percent suffer persistent PCS lasting more than three months or even years through the rest of their lives. Among the many symptoms are headaches, nausea or vomiting, fatigue, sensitivity to noise and light, depression, difficulty sleeping, and poor concentration and memory.

Diagnosis and treatment of PCS in children is a critical issue that has divided physicians and researchers—to the detriment of children. Leaving the condition untreated, or misdiagnosed as psychological or emotional issues, puts the child at a significant disadvantage, struggling with symptoms that can directly impact their development and lifelong performance and achievements.

We wondered, *Would HBOT be successful for children as we had demonstrated for adults?* The answer was yes, but it took six years to complete the studies that in 2022 demonstrated HBOT's value for healing children with concussions.

Why so long? Because this study was for a pediatric population, it took us a year to get approval from Israel's Ministry of Health ethics committee. Recruiting participants for the study was a much bigger challenge. We had anticipated, with the ethical committee approval in hand, electronic medical records would lead us to thousands of children diagnosed as suffering from PCS. But the actual number was negligible. Why? Was it possible there was little or no PCS in children? We were incredulous. To find the answer, we had to initiate another study, which we will get to shortly.

The second challenge was to convince the parents to include their children in the HBOT study. Parents who had read about the highly positive outcomes from PCS studies with adults already published were enthusiastic initially.

"It's clear to me that if it's working on adults, it will work on children," many told us. "I want to get the treatment for my child. I will even pay for it." Our study included a placebo control group, but parents resisted committing to a new three-month clinical study without our assurance the child would, in fact, receive the HBOT treatment and not the placebo.

We could not reveal whether a child would be in the group receiving the treatments or the control group. That would violate standards for random-controlled clinical studies. Yet many parents could not accept the odds that they might bring their child to the hospital on sixty different days for the study sessions without the child receiving the actual HHP benefits from the fluctuating pressure and oxygen concentration in the chamber. Eventually, after recruiting a smaller group of twenty-five children with parents' approval through the help of pediatricians and other colleagues, we began.

Because stem cells in children are more sensitive to stimulation, we modified the protocol so that participants breathed 100 percent oxygen through a mask at 1.5 ATA instead of 2 ATA and for sixty

minutes instead of ninety. Otherwise, the study mirrored adult protocols with sixty daily HBOT sessions, five sessions per week over a
three-month period. Participants in the placebo or sham group
breathed normal air at 1.1 ATA for the first five minutes, then pressure
gradually was lowered. The slightly elevated pressure at the beginning
of the sham sessions was sufficient with the noise of the air flow to
create a true placebo effect by producing a "pop" in their ears to equal-
ize pressure in the middle ear.

The results: HBOT induced significant improvement in memory,
cognitive, and executive functions. Specific PCS symptoms that
improved included emotional scores, behavioral issues such as hyperactivity, and abilities to plan and organize activities.[9]

Along with the treatment group's significant clinical improvement,
MRIs showed correlating positive changes in areas of the cortex associated with PCS symptoms, leading to significant improvements in
measurements for memory, verbal fluency, and executive function. In
contrast to the treatment group, there were no improvements in the
baseline scores of participants in the placebo/sham group.

Errors in Diagnosing a Child's Post-Concussion Symptoms Should Stop

As I noted before, we wondered why we weren't finding children in
Israel with diagnoses of PCS. TBI is one of the most common reasons
children are taken to emergency rooms, a frequency averaging 150 to
400 of every 100,000 child ER visits. These visits came typically after
car accidents, falls from bicycles, blunt force trauma, and sports-related
head injuries.

Physicians in emergency rooms might consider a serious head
injury when they assessed a child. But the child usually was released
to the care of a primary physician when CT or MRI images indicated

no significant noticeable brain damage that needed further attention at that time in the hospital.

We couldn't guess at how often this might occur, so we initiated another clinical trial to seek an answer. PCS symptoms were evaluated in children eight to fifteen years old between six and sixty months after they were admitted to the emergency department in our hospital because of mTBI. The control group was composed of children of the same age range who also had been admitted to the emergency department but with a different diagnosis, a broken arm near the wrist known medically as an uncomplicated distal radius fracture.

The results demonstrated that approximately one in every four children brought to emergency rooms suffered from PCS, yet *none* was diagnosed with this brain injury by their caring physicians over time. The more common diagnosis cited one or more of these issues: concentration or learning problems, ADHD, memory problems, chronic migraines or other headaches, depression, sleep disorder, fatigue, and other adaptive disorders. Essentially, no one made the connection between the head injury and post-concussion symptoms. Going by available health records in Israel, you'd conclude children did not suffer concussions!

"The goal of evaluations in emergency rooms is to determine whether a child has a serious brain injury that needs immediate attention," says my colleague Eran Kozer, MD, head of emergency room services at Shamir Medical Center. "Unfortunately, based on how most medical systems operate today, we are missing the long-term follow-up of those children who in the emergency room did not have any observable motor dysfunction."

Current guidelines for treating concussion injuries only span the first two weeks of symptoms. For children with a misdiagnosed concussion, these medical errors can be tragic. Leaving the condition untreated puts the child at a significant disadvantage and directly impacts their development into adulthood. A Canadian study of nearly

450,000 children aged five to eighteen concluded that concussion is the number one risk factor for children who develop mental health issues, psychiatric hospitalization, or harm themselves.[10]

Knowing when post-concussion symptoms begin can make a huge difference. "The impacts from any brain injury during childhood will continue through the rest of that child's life. We must be more alert to any trauma that may have long-term consequences on our children's brains," says Dr. Uri Balla, director of the pediatric emergency room in Israel's Kaplan Medical Center and another of my colleagues on this study. "The loss of any brain functionality will prevent a child from fulfilling their potential in school, university, and social life."

Since our analysis showing widespread misdiagnosis of the post-concussions was published early in 2022,[11] we have urged caring physicians, especially pediatricians, to recommend high-resolution metabolic imaging of the brain such as SPECT or functional MRI as well as computerized neurocognitive testing by specialists as part of their follow-up evaluations of children who suffer from persistent symptoms even after minor concussions. Once we can see the damage in a brain injury, we can find the best way to treat it.

Concussion and Metabolic Dysfunction

In demonstrating that most patients suffering with PCS after a mild-to-moderate concussion have an area, or areas, of metabolic dysfunction in their brain, we had achieved a clearer insight into a misunderstood disease—an insight that would shape our future research with HBOT on other neurological brain injuries.

The next step, which Shir Daphna-Tekoah urged us to take as a concussion patient and then joined as an absolutely essential expert in childhood sexual trauma, was to investigate HBOT and fibromyalgia.

As we will see in the next chapter, my mother was a major factor as well in our decision to take that path.

Key Takeaways

1. Traumatic brain injury (TBI) is a leading cause of death and disability in the United States, with an estimated average of 1.4 million cases per year.
2. Brain regions with reduced blood/oxygen supply and diminished metabolism can recover much of their lost potency through HBOT. The clinical improvement is correlated with specific regions of the brain.
3. In children, the diagnosis of persistent post-concussion syndrome (PPCS) is largely dismissed. In a study completed in 2022, HBOT proved to be as beneficial for children with PPCS as it is for adults. Leaving the condition untreated puts the child at a significant disadvantage and directly impacts their whole life course.

CHAPTER 7

Fibromyalgia

We were only a month into the post-concussion syndrome study, but Shir Daphna-Tekoah was certain that the disabling pains, fatigue, headaches, extreme sensitivity to touch, and other symptoms that gripped her after the Revadim train disaster were already easing.

"Something was happening to my body," she remembers. "After the accident I had been too weak to even hold my six-month-old son, at just fifteen pounds. I was full of pain. Now, I felt less pain and had more strength. He was four years old, more than forty pounds, and I could pick him up and look into his eyes."

Shir was convinced the early metabolic effects of our HBOT sessions were calming her previously diagnosed fibromyalgia symptoms *in addition to* the brain fog, memory loss, and other post-concussion symptoms that she and other participants had been screened for in this study.

"Shai, this is a phenomenon," she told me. I wasn't sure, not yet, but Shir was a brilliant scientist with exceptional academic credentials now shaping insights into her intensely personal medical condition. "We have to research this, too," she said.

Explaining Fibromyalgia

As much as 5 percent of the general population worldwide is believed to suffer from fibromyalgia, and most, by a huge factor, are women.[1] Women are nine times more likely to be afflicted by fibromyalgia pain than men.[2] Symptoms include chronic widespread pain above and below the waist, fatigue, restless or nonrestorative sleep, and extreme sensitivity to touch. There is also brain fog that curbs mental functions required to think and reason clearly.

The biological setbacks involve damage to the normal metabolic functions in the areas of the brain responsible for interpreting signals from the body.[3] It is as if the brain is sounding a fire alarm, yet there is no fire. Until recently, many rheumatologists—physicians who specialize in joints, autoimmune diseases, and soft tissues—routinely dismissed patients' complaints of "hurting all over," because they could not locate inflammation or any other physical signs that could help in diagnosing a medical problem. "It's all in your mind," patients were told.

Despite rapid progress this century in describing the metabolic malfunctioning in fibromyalgia, some physicians continue to do this, unfortunately. A dismissive reply is quite common in France, for example. I know because many patients from there come to Israel for treatment. Some of these patients are even *physicians*!

We know now that fibromyalgia symptoms originate in the brain, in pathways of regions responsible for interpreting sensations coming from the body. In the past decade, the term *central sensitization syndrome* has gained credence as a catchall phrase for this malfunction. Fibromyalgia is a prototype of the syndrome. Moreover, medical scientists have shown that chronic pain syndromes, and fibromyalgia in particular, evolve over a lifetime.[4] This finding confirmed that the central nervous system itself can evolve and rewire even after it is fully developed.

Knowing this, we speculated after the successful clinical studies on stroke and post-concussion syndrome that the HHP might heal fibromyalgia symptoms as well. These ailments, we concluded, might reflect wounds hidden in the brain, wounds that might have occurred as far back as early childhood and never healed.

Brain damage in fibromyalgia might be related to injuries from a car accident or a fall—some blow to the head. We call this a *mechanical brain injury*. Or the damage might have been caused by viruses that infected the nerve system. Both culminate in biological injuries with mental consequences. Yet, as we discovered in our fibromyalgia studies, the pain might be caused by some previous severe emotional stress, such as childhood sexual abuse or molestation.

This is a key point: *psychology can determine biology.*

And vice versa: biological injury can manifest initially through symptoms of psychological distress.

Frida Kahlo: Self-Portraits, Severe Pain

The celebrated Mexican painter Frida Kahlo suffered a concussion in a bus accident in her late teens, plus a broken spine that kept her in traction for months.

During the 1930s and '40s, moving through her most prolific creative periods, accumulating what ultimately would be fifty-five self-portraits, she continued to endure intense pain. That pain, as well as her determination to persevere in the face of it, dominates many of these arresting autobiographical visions.

Here is Frida in a wooded setting, her stoic face painted on the head of a large deer buck, nine long piercing arrows drawing blood along its back, chest, and neck (*The Wounded Deer*, 1946). There is Frida, teardrops staining her cheeks, nails tacked into her naked arms, breasts, chest, face, and neck, her torso cleaved to expose a rigid steel column supplanting spinal vertebrae (*The Broken Column*, 1944). And here again is Frida, a black cat peering ahead from one shoulder, a preoccupied spider monkey on the other. The monkey tugs lightly on a necklace of thorns that grips her neck and entraps her shoulders and chest (*Self-portrait with Thorn Necklace and Hummingbird*, 1940).

Did Frida Kahlo, who died at age forty-seven in 1954, have fibromyalgia? The diagnosis was unknown during her lifetime. Yet looking at what we know of her difficult medical history and frank journal entries, and awestruck by her stunning artistic legacy, the answer most certainly must be yes.

Shir, My Mother, and the Urgency for a Clinical Study

For two years, Shir had been studying the links between psychological trauma and fibromyalgia symptoms many people in the train disaster had developed. That medical research was led by Dan Buskila, an Israeli rheumatologist whose earlier studies helped establish in medical journals globally that fibromyalgia is a serious physical illness.[5]

Intellectually, I didn't need convincing. The cause–effect connection between trauma and fibromyalgia symptoms emerged in my own mother not long before I became aware of Shir and some other participants in the concussion study reporting a release from their fibromyalgia symptoms. Remember, we had not screened any of these participants for fibromyalgia.

My mother, Allis Efrati, had been an excellent student as a teenager, but after one of her brothers died tragically in a farm accident, she was so shaken that she was forced to abandon her high school studies. Some years later, her trauma was compounded when her other brother died unexpectedly from a hepatitis infection.

Decades later, in her sixties, she complained to me that her persistent pains were worsening, taking a heavier toll all over her body. She tired easily and was not thinking clearly. I examined her but failed to identify any "pure" physical problem. One day, I saw her recoil suddenly, her face etched in awful pain, after reaching out to hug one of my daughters. *She can't be imaging this*, I thought. *The pain must be biologically real. She is really debilitated.*

Images of the cross-sectional brain scans showed what I had expected: my mother had brain damage. The brain SPECT images showed irregular metabolism in the areas that interpret pain. In other words, neurons there were misfiring. With the results of our HBOT stroke study still fresh in mind, I knew immediately, "I can fix this."

As she journeyed through sixty days of HBOT sessions, my mother's pains subsided, and then vanished. "My dear son. You must do for others what you have done for me!" she implored.

I felt overburdened and a bit weary at the time and had no scientific interest in fibromyalgia beyond my delight in HBOT's success in peeling away my mother's symptoms. I was overseeing the hyperbarics and concussions study, managing care for nephrology patients, assembling the talent and agenda for the new Sagol Center for Hyperbaric Medicine and Research, and teaching medical students and residents as a professor at Tel Aviv University.

But then, as Shir and other participants in the concussion study reported fading fibromyalgia symptoms, I realized the potential scope and urgency of the matter. Plus, when your mother asks you to do something, you must do it. I laid plans with my team to organize a random-controlled clinical study of HBOT treatments for fibromyalgia patients to follow the concussion study. In time, we would add a second clinical study focused solely on one set of fibromyalgia patients: women who were in psychotherapy counseling for childhood sexual abuse.

A Terrifying Reprise of Childhood Sexual Abuse

Our first clinical study of fibromyalgia involved a random group of forty patients—and it was a jarring event for me personally. Repressed childhood memories surfaced unexpectedly for three women during the first phase of the treatments—horrible, visual, *and* visceral revivals of childhood sexual abuse. I was unprepared, frightened as well. We never thought something like this could happen.

What *was* happening?

Our memories are catalogued and mainly—but not always—retrieved in regions of the cortex. If we experience a searingly painful event that is incompatible with our perception, our brains are conditioned to respond with a kind of amnesia to protect us from vivid recurring memories of that event, or even being conscious of it at all. The effect is a neurological breakdown. Our ability to orderly connect aspects of memory, identity, perception, and consciousness involved in storing memories is severely degraded. In medical terms, the brain is "dissociating" the work of those different functions required to catalogue a normal healthy memory.

Without doubt, childhood sexual abuse is an exceptionally severe example of emotional and physical trauma that triggers dissociation.

The memory of the specific traumatic experience is neither permanently lost nor forgotten, yet it becomes unavailable in our conscious minds for a period that may last decades or even a lifetime.

This "chronic dysregulation" can lead to long-standing neurobiological troubles that resemble, or even overlap, those we described in chapter 6 that are common in patients with PCS due to a traumatic brain injury.

Repetitive trauma inflicted by a relative or close relation often happens to children in cases of sexual abuse. Unable to escape these attacks physically, the traumatized child disengages psychologically, dissociating as much as possible. As this happens, certain areas of the brain involved in normal perception are disconnected.

Physiologically, during dissociation, blood vessels constrict and normal blood flows and oxygen supplies can decline so seriously that those areas of the brain that normally would store the memory become dormant. The memory becomes repressed, inaccessible. As we have seen, however, functional brain scans enable us to determine activity in a specific, low-performing brain region we are treating with the HHP by measuring blood flows. Flows will increase in newly active, healing brain regions as they decline in healthy areas with less clinical need.

As we discovered with great alarm in that first fibromyalgia clinical study, these areas can be reactivated by the HBOT protocol, resurfacing those dormant memories as the regions once disabled by metabolic breakdowns begin to recover their normal function.

Once we first witnessed that stunning resurfacing of those repressed memories, we quickly brought in psychotherapy counselors to reassure these newly traumatized patients: those resurfacing memories were from events long ago. One of my first urgent calls went to Shir before dawn one day. She was an expert in childhood sexual abuse and, as a participant in the post-concussion study, she had experienced personally and understood medically the evolving physiological changes along the regimen of HBOT sessions.

She immediately helped me grasp what was happening: the first month of HBOT treatments in the fibromyalgia study had begun to restore normal memory functions in areas of these women's brains that had been largely shut down, but not lost, after traumatic shock from the abuse.

We acted to assure these women that they were in a safe place now. In those intense exchanges, we then learned and later verified that they had suffered psychological stress wounds as children, wounds invisible to our eyes as physicians, but they were wounds nonetheless. Those biological brain wounds never healed. The "storage memories" could not be accessed until the wounds were repaired by HHP.

HBOT and Trauma of Childhood Sexual Abuse

Our first fibromyalgia study had uncovered the unexpected terrors of childhood sexual abuse that nine women participating in the study had experienced. Would a treatment combining HBOT and psychotherapy heal those brain wounds that we believed were at the root of the sensory sensitivity pains triggered for fibromyalgia? The answer was yes.

Those nine women, with their dramatic improvement, motivated us to initiate another fibromyalgia study, this time focused on a subgroup of patients whose trauma from childhood sexual abuse we speculated had created the brain wounds responsible for their fibromyalgia symptoms.

One of the world's leading researchers in assessing, validating, and alleviating childhood trauma through drawings, dance, music, and other creative arts, Rachel Lev-Wiesel, was a vital contributor on our team of investigators.

A fibromyalgia sufferer herself her entire life, Rachel was the first candidate to sign up for the original fibromyalgia study. Shir had described to her how her own HBOT sessions during the mild traumatic brain injury (mTBI) study erased her concussion and fibromyalgia symptoms. Shir was one of Rachel's doctoral students in clinical social work at Ben Gurion University.

Participating in that subsequent first fibromyalgia study "changed my life," Rachel says. She was sixty-two years old at the time. "I had more energy. I slept much better. The pains in my legs went away. I could walk up stairs without breathing so heavily."

She quickly urged me to organize a related clinical study: treating fibromyalgia patients who had been traumatized by sexual abuse when they were children. Her concept was to support the full sessions of hyperbaric chamber treatments through the three months and beyond with counseling by psychotherapists.

"If HBOT works on the brain, maybe this will help with psychological trauma, with childhood sexual abuse, and other forms of abuse," she told me. She had learned by then, after more than thirty years of research and counseling with child abuse victims, especially of sexual molestation, that most of these abuse victims have fibromyalgia symptoms. "Okay, let's do a pre-test and see what happens," I replied.

All the usual measures we applied after the study—brain scans, metabolic functions, questionnaires, and so on—confirmed that all five abuse survivors with fibromyalgia that Rachel recruited recovered at least 80 percent of their damaged brain capacities. In some cases, they recovered *all* those functions.

This was an exciting outcome, yet I was still cautious. "Let's do a second pre-test with five more," I said.

When we validated the same remarkable results from HBOT for those second five patients, I was convinced. Rachel took a lead role for this second study. We initially explored recruiting only adolescents up to age eighteen who had been sexually abused in boarding schools. We wanted to demonstrate (with before and after brain scans) both the damage from the abuse trauma and the healing with HBOT sessions. But limiting the study to adolescents raised legitimate ethical concerns, so we restricted the study to women between ages eighteen and sixty-five who had been sexually abused. The brain scan objective was not abandoned; an eighteen-year-old's brain structure is quite similar to that of a sixteen-year-old's.

Helping Young Abuse Victims Defend Themselves

Fewer than 10 percent of children who have been molested tell anyone about the abuse. The more severe the abuse, the more reluctant children are to talk about it. They are especially reluctant to open up and describe their fears to social workers, physicians and other medical professionals, court investigators, or others with whom they have had little or no prior contact.

"Children cannot disclose, they cannot articulate the abuse they experienced, especially to strangers," says Rachel Lev-Wiesel, professor emeritus in social work at the University of Haifa. She has published more than 200 papers and seven books in her forty years researching and counseling child abuse victims. "It is like asking them to walk when they have broken bones."

As a result, nearly 90 percent of childhood sexual abuse criminal cases in Israel are closed without any charges made against suspected perpetrators. Still worse, and horrifying: roughly two-thirds of these cases are dismissed due to lack of evidence; victimized children are sent back into the hands of a parent or other family member suspected of abuse, and the children are silenced.

Often, fathers persuade a court in custody dispute cases that the mother is attempting to alienate a child from the father by inventing false allegations for the child about specific instances of sexual abuse. In these high-conflict cases, allegations of sexual abuse usually are dismissed, with the father given rights either to joint custody or full custody of the child.

Yet children as young as six years old can and do express graphic scenes of sexual abuse in sketches that have been accepted by courts. "You cannot implant elaborate pornographic scene images in the minds of young children. They are able to bypass their dissociation from a traumatic event to draw what really happened," Rachel says. In some cases, children are able to create these drawings in a courtroom before a judge.

Rachel teaches those and other skills for helping young abuse victims defend themselves from predators to her students, psychotherapists, social workers, lawyers, and legal staff at the Emili Sagol Center for Creative Arts Therapies, a world-renowned center she directs at the University of Haifa. She has consulted on hundreds of child abuse cases in the United States, Europe, and Asia, as well as Israel.

One of Rachel's motivations for seeking to initiate a clinical study including adolescents for the second fibromyalgia study had been to influence criminal courts to accept advanced metabolic brain scans as evidence of biological damage inflicted on a child by a suspected perpetrator. Another is to persuade state agencies to provide HBOT treatments and psychotherapy to help every child recover from sexual abuse.

We are optimistic that these changes will happen over time. Meanwhile, Rachel tapped foundation grants to support parents eager to have their children receive HBOT in addition to psychotherapy treatments.

One set of parents, a judge and a lawyer, immediately seized the opportunity. Their fifteen-year-old daughter, molested by a grandfather when she was between the ages of six and eight, had struggled through years of morose, silent behavior, refusing counseling, not completing any school assignments, temper outbursts, and several attempts to injure herself.

A few months after the HBOT treatments and supporting psychotherapy, she transformed, becoming more engaging, with new focus and confidence. She committed to a college-preparatory track of studies in biotechnology. Within months she was named her school's most outstanding student, posting a grade average of ninety-five across all her courses.

She became eager to tell her story publicly, to anyone in a position to help others struggling, withdrawn, and desperate like she had been for half her childhood. Speaking before lawyers at a Sagol Center conference in 2023, she urged them to support a new law that would enable any sexual abuse victim to receive the treatment she did. "I never believed I could become again the girl I was before (the abuse) happened," she said. "I feel I have fully recovered."

Thirty women aged eighteen or older with fibromyalgia participated in the second clinical study; fifteen in the treatment group and another fifteen in the control group. All had received psychotherapy counseling for at least a year before joining the study. Their fibromyalgia was induced by their history with childhood sexual abuse, most often by an immediate family member or family acquaintance.

They had failed to make much if any progress in alleviating their symptoms from the two medications prescribed by their therapists, duloxetine (Cymbalta) and pregabalin (Lyrica), that had been approved for treating fibromyalgia in addition to psychotherapy and physical therapy, and other remedies also recommended by physicians. HBOT would be the first attempt for them to heal malfunctioning brain tissue with a biological treatment designed to regenerate the tissue's normal, pre-injury activity.

"One problem survivors of child sexual abuse have is a disintegration between body and soul," Rachel says. "In their minds, they feel that the body betrayed them by collaborating with the perpetrator of the abuse. For children, the perpetrator is the only one who can release them from the extreme sexual arousal they experienced even long after the episode has ended. In that way, they become dependent on the perpetrator."

The self-hatred that follows can spark suicidal thoughts—even attempts. "It's like somebody comes to your house when you are not there and starts doing whatever they want in your drawers, your rooms, everything," she says. "I call it 'soul homelessness'; a dislocation of the soul from the body. You don't feel safe in that house anymore."

Rachel had the foresight to ask patients to keep a daily journal during their HBOT treatment for months in addition to what we had planned for standard medical follow-up and brain imaging. The patients were encouraged to create drawings in their journals to express feelings, thoughts, and memories.

Patients in the treatment group of this HBOT, fibromyalgia, and childhood sexual abuse study had significant improvement in all parameters we evaluated related to their fibromyalgia and PTSD. Moreover, 53 percent in the HBOT group recovered to the point where their symptoms no longer met the criteria for a diagnosis of fibromyalgia syndrome. That compared with only 6.7 percent in the control group before these participants were crossed over to receive the HBOT treatment.[6]

Rachel has spoken about these studies before hundreds of colleagues at conferences in Israel and thousands in the United States and East Asia. She says, "Professionals in social work around the world know more and more that HBOT should be combined with psychotherapy. Those whose clients come for HBOT sessions and continue with psychotherapy say they wouldn't have believed before how many of their clients' mental blocks were removed. Many survivors no longer need medicines, or even psychotherapy."

Today, more than 70 percent of all fibromyalgia patients completing the HBOT protocols we administer at our clinics improve to levels where they no longer meet the criteria for fibromyalgia diagnosis.

Phase I: Terrifying Memories Resurface

One woman, Berniece, age fifty-three, described a terrifying repressed memory with visions and visceral disgust of being molested and raped repeatedly by classmates when she was fourteen. The flashbacks during the treatment sessions often started with unbearable sexual arousal accompanied by shortness of breath and other symptoms of panic attacks.

"I can't understand how I, or anyone else for that matter, could forget such experiences," she wrote later in the journal she kept for a

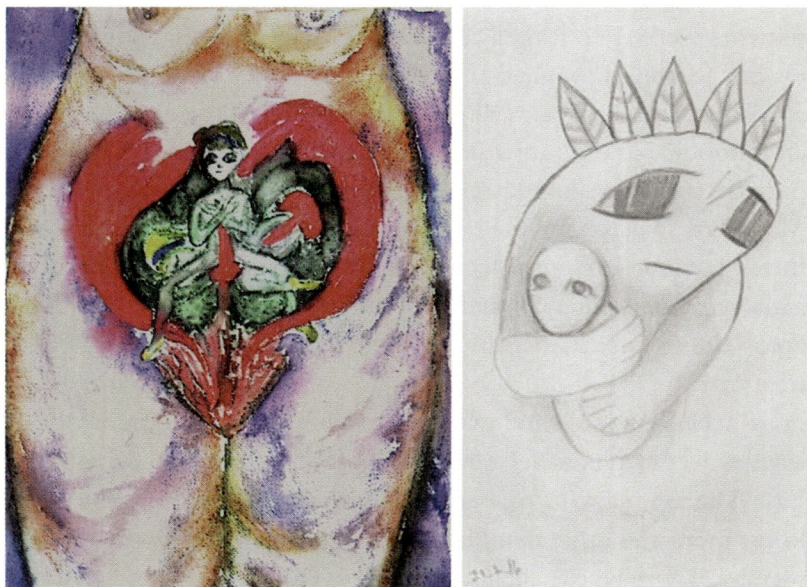

Figures 7-1 (left) and 7-2 (right): These drawings were created by two participants, ages fifty-three and twenty-four, in the first phase of their HBOT. The drawings graphically reveal emotions of distress, fear, sadness, and entrapment. The traumatic sexual abuse event seems apparent in the first drawing (Figure 7-1, left) by Berniece. She had been molested and raped by classmates when she was fourteen. The little girl in the second drawing (Figure 7-2, right), created by Miriam, is caught by some kind of monster. Miriam had been sexually abused as a child by a family member.

post-treatment therapy session. Yet, Berniece went on, "I continued to function as an excellent student. I focused on my dancing. I avoided peer gatherings, rationalizing this avoidance to myself and my parents as 'lack of interest' and 'will to excel.'"

Another participant, Miriam, twenty-four, reported unbearable pain in her abdomen, "as if someone is stabbing me with a knife."* These symptoms were followed by the surfacing of new memories of the abuse, which revealed further abuse by her mother.

These new, vivid, coherent, and detailed memories altered the narratives Miriam had carried about her mother and her childhood. Those memories of abuse by her mother had not surfaced before the HBOT, nor during psychotherapy given before the dual treatment. A day before the dissociated memory emerged, she had written "I can't breathe, I am so physically stressed, tensed, shaking from within, as if I have a volcano in my throat that is going to burst any minute, I shut my lips so hard, I feel as if I am burning from within, but no one sees. My body responds as if in delay, tensed, anxious. I feel as if memory is stuck in my lower back . . . a flashback that only the body remembers . . . the brain does not. My poor body is shaking and not breathing . . ."

Phase II: More Self-Compassion; Less Horror, Fear, or Disgust

In the second phase, between HBOT sessions twenty-one and forty, patients reported fewer sleeping difficulties and disturbances. Nightmares vanished. Participants described this as the soothing phase. With these changes, they began to feel better physically. In the oxygen chamber, they often fell asleep or said they felt as though they had been meditating or were in, as one woman reported, "a floating state."

---

* Patient names here have been changed to protect their privacy.

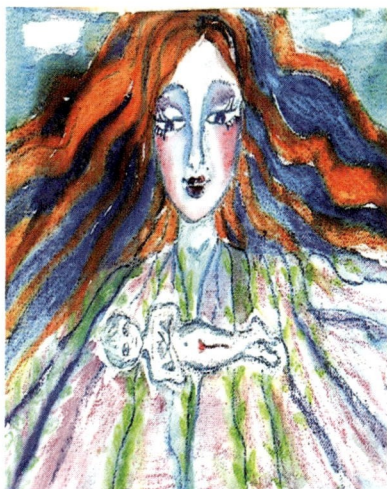

Figure 7-3: A drawing Berniece made during the second phase of HBOT reveals a sense of relaxation and safety, even optimism. The inside figure lies, as if floating, in the chest-stomach area.

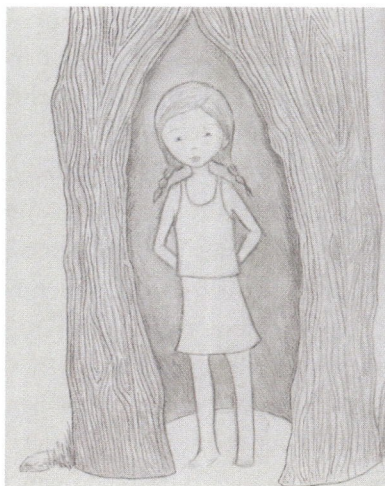

Figure 7-4: In this second drawing by Miriam, the young girl is protected by a tree trunk, yet she is open to the world. Although she seems not ready yet to hold out her hands, she can see and be seen by the world.

Physical pains abated. Feelings of sorrow or self-compassion rose, and old ones of horror, fear, or disgust faded.

Phase III: Dramatic Improvement

In the last phase, between sessions forty-one and sixty, women described a dramatic improvement in physical and emotional symptoms. As the symptoms dissolved, they recovered. They reported a surge in energy and a new confidence in their ability to enjoy life and think creatively about what they would like to achieve and do. For them, the past no longer was physically active in the present: "The past has become the past." They envisioned an exciting new future, free of past burdens.

Hostile attitudes toward the people who abused them, ambivalent feelings of love and hate, or of fear and longing, dissipated into indifference. "Today my door is closed to those who tried to hurt me. I chose," one woman, Grace, wrote in a poetic cadence. "I am not surprised but rather aware of the harms and injuries. I breathe deeply into the pain, know how to soothe it, calm my soul. This is not related to the others; my wound became my own. Today others can no longer hurt me, perhaps only remind me of the past hurt."

For Grace, as for many participants whose repressed memories of childhood traumas resurfaced during phase one, the past had become the past during the third set of twenty daily sessions, phase three. It was like having an abscess evacuated. Repressed memories surfaced, but patients were reassured: You are doing bereavement of the past. You are not in the same environment where you suffered as a child. Your world now is safe.

"I hear the birds, I listen to street noises, I hear myself," another participant wrote during this phase. "For the first time, I notice that there are colors other than just black and white in the world . . . I even discovered that I have green eyes; I always thought that they were black."

"I broke into uncontrolled weeping at the beginning of the HBOT treatment," another woman wrote. "Slowly, and with daily accompaniment of writing and meaningful therapy sessions, the memories were cast into

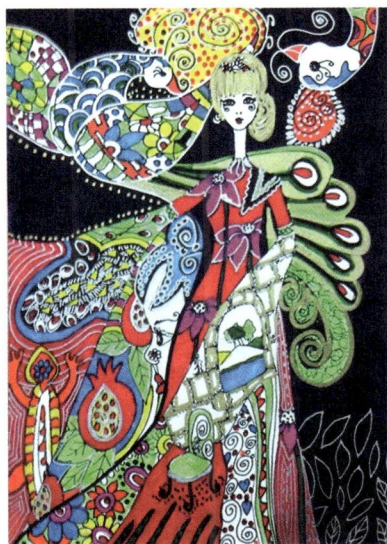

Figure 7-5. A drawing by Berniece during the third phase of HBOT.

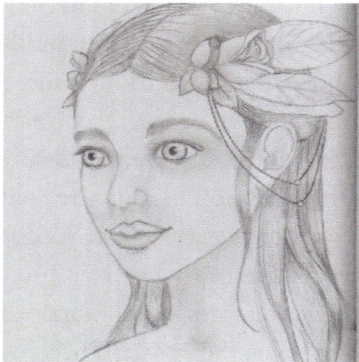

Figure 7-6. A drawing created
by Miriam during the third phase.

words and drawings. I could shed layer after layer: weightiness, depression, anxiety, helplessness, denial, and numbness. I am happy to say today that everything changed for me, how I look, the way I perceive myself, the way I cope with hardships, the life I would like to lead. I used to be afraid of losing control; I feel I gained control over myself."

A Third Head-Injury Study: HBOT Compared with Medications

We are treating a wound with HBOT. When the wound tissue regenerates, the symptoms disappear. A tissue is a tissue.

Fibromyalgia patients whose symptoms were triggered by a concussion related to some mechanical incident are relatively easier to treat in contrast to patients with psychological trauma, such as childhood sexual abuse. Car crashes and falls are frequent causes of concussions.

In those cases, we have a clear medical issue, an insult. We need to repair biologically the damaged brain tissue that is responsible for analyzing signals coming from the body, in addition to treating any psychological disruptions related to the incident. For Shir Daphna-Tekoah, for example, the incident was a train disaster. Our HBOT treatments in these cases focus mostly on alleviating symptoms of general pain and cognitive decline that we see in most cases.

An HBOT clinical study we mounted in October 2017 at the Sagol Center demonstrated that a group of twenty-nine fibromyalgia patients recovered more broadly and extensively after the full three months of

HBOT sessions than a comparable group of twenty-nine patients in the study. That latter group was treated with two medications approved by the FDA for fibromyalgia and most widely prescribed in Israel—duloxetine and pregabalin.

Results for patients in the HBOT treatment group were superior in every dimension we measured: reduction of pain intensity, quality of life, and emotional and social function. After the treatment, 37 percent no longer had symptoms associated with a fibromyalgia diagnosis; none in the medication group had come that far. Brain imaging with SPECT showed sharp improvements in oxygen supply into areas of the brain whose metabolic recovery closely correlated with weakened or entirely resolved symptoms.

These brain areas included the anterior temporal lobe (repository for recalling specific knowledge of objects, people, words, and facts), the prefrontal cortex (regulates complex cognitive, emotional, and behavior functions), and the perirhinal cortex (involved in both visual perception and memory, part of a larger system for assigning meaning to objects).

The imaging results underscored the important role the central nervous system has in the causes of fibromyalgia.

What about Military PTSD?

Childhood sexual abuse is a post-traumatic stress disorder, a PTSD that we classify as a civilian PTSD. What about PTSD carried by millions of military veterans, known as military PTSD? Our studies with these courageous women who confronted and silenced their buried memories of abuse gave us new visions for how HBOT might reduce or erase military veterans' PTSD symptoms.

Our ongoing research and success in healing military veterans with PTSD brain injuries, which we'll turn to next, have shown this indeed is the case.

Key Takeaways

1. Fibromyalgia symptoms include chronic widespread pain above and below the waist, fatigue, restless or non-restorative sleep, and extreme sensitivity to touch. Also, brain fog curbs mental functions required to think and reason clearly.

2. Brain damage in fibromyalgia might be related to injuries from a car accident or a fall (some blow to the head), viruses that infected the nerve system, surgery with general anesthesia, a traumatic event, or severe emotional stress.

3. Chronic pain syndromes and fibromyalgia in particular evolve throughout our lifetime; the central nervous system itself can evolve and re-wire after it is fully developed.

CHAPTER 8

Post-Traumatic Stress Disorder (PTSD)

Growing up, I was an excellent student with high grades and, as I later discovered, a photographic memory.

When I was in my third and fourth years of high school, I thought it a waste of my time to spend hours in class where teachers who were not experts in a subject reviewed and explained textbook material. Going to class seemed silly. I didn't understand why a teacher covered something you could read and understand by yourself at home.

Ah, I thought, *instead of going to class I can earn money tutoring other students in physics and math.* I especially loved physics and felt certain that was where my professional future would lie. Many students found those subjects difficult and frustrating, and I did have the privilege to teach them.

After high school, I went into the military, as most everyone does in Israel—a commitment of three years or longer if you want to be a career soldier. I was a paratrooper. The time in the military was tough, but I believed then as I do now that if it does not break you, it builds you. In my case it was "growing time."

I was a good navigator, especially at night when you cannot open and read a map. My photographic memory enabled me to recall accurate details of any map. I didn't have to memorize, for example, having to move a hundred meters in one direction at one landmark, then a hundred meters in another direction. I could look at a map during the day and remember the picture of the map. If my patrol needed to navigate somewhere at night, I had the map details in my head.

Those years marked my first encounters with dangerous blast (explosion) and traumatic brain injuries (TBIs) and PTSD.

During Israel's Second Lebanon War in the summer of 2006, I re-enlisted as a reservist, a paratrooper again, as I had been during active duty in my late teens and early twenties. I was a physician now, serving in a different role. This opened me to new experiences and insights in treating combat and training injuries—a specialty known as military medicine.

During this war, and especially after it, I needed to confront biases I had held about the symptoms and struggles with PTSD that torment many soldiers and veterans stemming from what we call *military-related PTSD*.

After the war I stayed in touch with my combat team. These are some of the best friends I have. A few confided that they were not sleeping at night, not able to go back to work or maintain a steady daily routine. They complained about emotional things. I was certain these were psychological hurdles, something they could defeat with their willpower and a strength of character that I once knew.

And I was dismissive: "The war is over. We had the fight. Your hands and legs are okay. You are alive, and you're breathing. You don't have any physical injury. So, what the hell is going on with you? Get back to life—and that's it."

My view was shared by many people then in medicine and society broadly. The consensus was PTSD is a psychological setback, perhaps even a personality flaw. I had no interest medically in PTSD. The field was all questionnaires and wide-ranging opinions. I had no time for patients worried their lives were being consumed. I was arrogant. There were no effective scientific ways to diagnose, measure, and treat those symptoms. "PTSD? You can see my wife. She's a social worker. I don't deal with that emotional stuff."

Correcting My Faulty Conclusions

My churlish attitude began to change a few years later as I examined those brain scans from our first fibromyalgia study. *Wow. Maybe my perspective on PTSD is wrong*, I thought. *Might PTSD also be a brain injury triggered by psychological trauma? If so, might HBOT help heal that biological injury as well, just as we had confirmed for fibromyalgia?*

Around the same time, three unrelated events convinced me that I needed to answer those questions.

I knew about a military hero in Israel, a fighter in one of the elite forces, whose life had fallen apart in the years after his discharge. He had lost his marriage and family, his small business, and then a series of jobs as an employee. A brother who took him into his home soon discovered that this military veteran rarely slept, instead drinking heavily and keeping a light on all night in his room. Overwhelmed during his post-military descent by panic attacks and anxieties, he had been too ashamed to reveal these terrors to anyone or seek help. Was this a dramatic case of PTSD?

Next, a colleague was developing studies with rats that showed through vivid brain imaging what a PTSD injury looks like in the brain: a real biological injury. An HBOT regimen for those rats initiated after a carefully staged trauma event alleviated much of the biological damage. You could see actual biological damage, then healing, in images of the rats' brains taken before and after the treatments!

In the experiments, my colleague exposed rats for an hour in a small cage to litter soaked in cat urine; another group of rats was studied under the same conditions except the litter in their cages was unspoiled. The first group, trapped in that small space with an inescapable fear, suffered extreme psychological trauma.

That trauma, a pathological evaluation showed, had *injured* their brains.

She and I could see serious neuronal damage in the traumatized rats; the bright colors that illuminate healthy activity had darkened. Then, too, tests involving mazes and sudden startle sounds confirmed sharply higher anxiety behaviors that the research team had observed.

After seeing those before-and-after brain images and test results, I had to conclude: PTSD is a real brain wound, a biological event, not solely psychological and definitely not an indicator of character flaw. The next question: *Could HBOT also help human PTSD patients recover?*

The third push to study PTSD and HBOT came from a psychiatrist during one of our first conferences in Israel on hyperbarics and brain injuries. He had treated hundreds of PTSD patients.

"You know now that HBOT heals symptoms for stroke, concussion, and now fibromyalgia," he said to me privately. "PTSD is an epidemic in Israel, a huge social crisis. It disrupts the lives of thousands of combat veterans. If you can demonstrate that HBOT helps PTSD victims recover, it would be a major breakthrough."

A First Study with Israeli Military Veterans

The clinical study we mounted, from March 2018 to October 2019, was the first to focus solely on veterans whose PTSD diagnosis had been confirmed by Israel's Ministry of Defense. The results were convincing scientifically. They illustrated that HBOT helped reduce PTSD symptoms such as nightmares and flashbacks, rebuild damaged brain tissue, and restore healthy neuron functioning.

Ages of participants ranged from twenty-five to sixty years old; on average, they had left active military duty eleven years before. Half were treated with the full sixty sessions of HBOT over three months; the other half in a control group were given a placebo instead of HBOT during the same period.

Their symptoms had persisted despite at least a year of psychotherapy counseling and regular doses of prescribed medicines and whose last traumatic experience, a combat situation, was at least four years prior. In medical terms, we had screened for participants with PTSD symptoms who were "treatment resistant."

That is, we excluded anyone who had suffered a concussion from a blast injury, car crash, or mechanical accident, accepting only veterans who had emotional distress and post-traumatic symptoms. For them, psychotherapy and prescription drugs were of little or no help in calming symptoms.

We needed those guardrails to avoid criticism that any prior psychotherapy or medical treatments might have reduced the need for hyperbaric therapy as a first line of therapy, whatever the study results would be. For some patients, not many, a few months of psychotherapy does reduce or even erase their symptoms.

One key measure of HBOT's impact—a detailed psychiatric interview measuring frequency of nightmares, flashbacks, and other symptoms (known as the CAPS-V score)—showed dramatic change. The mean score of psychiatric issues cited by veterans declined by more than 30 percent in the treatment group (with no significant change in the placebo group).

The gains are more impressive when you appreciate how that psychiatric scorecard understates the magnitude of change. For

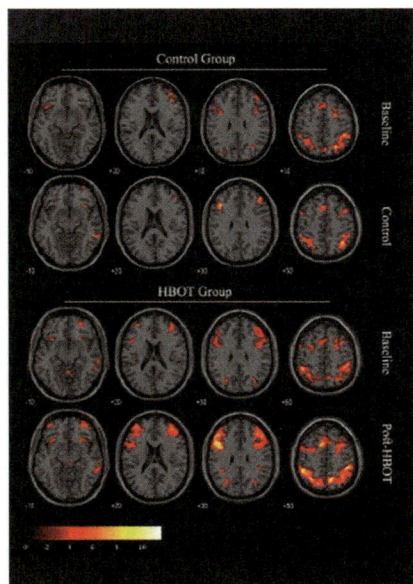

Figure 8-1

example, two nightmares a week counts as three points. Two nightmares a month counts as two points. That is more than a 75 percent drop in frequency of nightmares, but it equates to only one less point in the total score. In this study, the mean score declined by eighteen points overall, to twenty-eight from forty-six.

Another measure was brain images using functional MRI (fMRI) technologies. We asked veterans lying in an MRI machine to memorize a series of letters. Then, as they worked on the mental task, we evaluated how regions of their brains governing memory responded.

In these pictures (Figure 8-1), red regions mark the regions active as they performed the task. The contrasting images confirm that HBOT repaired damage to the frontal lobe region that regulates emotions (fronto-limbic circuit), and the hippocampus, which manages memory.

In medical terms, HBOT repaired the fronto-limbic integrity, with improved recruitment of the left dorsolateral pre-frontal cortex, of both thalami and of the left hippocampus. The thalami is comprised of two masses of gray matter between cerebral hemispheres. They orchestrate how we perceive sensory information, including pain.

Moreover, an MRI-DTI (magnetic resonance imaging and diffusion tensor tractography) evaluation showed improved microstructural integrity of neurons and tissue between the frontal and parietal or temporal regions. Among other roles, those regions govern cognitive skills such as concentrating and planning to achieve a goal. Damage can cause personality changes and impulsive responses to any unexpected stimuli.

Restoration of the fronto-limbic circuit may explain the significant improvement we registered for veterans in the HBOT group related to emotional regulations as reflected by the sharply improved CAPS-V score, in particular in reducing arousal and reactivity symptoms (E criterion of the CAPS-V data). Moreover, restoration of the fronto-limbic circuit may explain the significant decline of nightmares, flashbacks, and other intrusive symptoms reflected in the CAPS-V score (B criterion).

A strong connection between clinical and biological data is a holy grail in medical science studies. "A good correlation between clinical and brain function results means that the changes in brain activity are related to the clinical symptoms," notes Keren Doenyas-Barak, a physician at Shamir Medical Center and a leader of this study.

My Co-Author on This Chapter, Keren Doenyas-Barak

Keren Doenyas-Barak followed my career track into internal medicine and then nephrology studies after completing her medical degree in 2002, and she soon became one of the first research physicians to join my nephrology team at Shamir Medical Center. Like many physicians in nephrology, she had a particular interest in how the body's biology functions—its physiology.

She first joined our HBOT research team after seeing the unanticipated results of the stroke and concussion studies. She wondered if HBOT might be an effective treatment for patients with chronic kidney disease; namely, if HBOT could improve blood flows in the kidney.

The kidneys are one of the target organs damaged by atherosclerosis, the natural process that narrows flows within our blood vessels as we age chronologically. Diabetes, hypertension, smoking, and obesity all exacerbate atherosclerosis, and they significantly increase risks that a patient will lose kidney functions.

Keren's intuition as a physician and her sense of purpose were stirred further by the surprise surfacing of inaccessible memories of childhood sexual abuse in the first fibromyalgia study and those women's path to recovery. She wondered, *If HBOT could help these women recover from the pain symptoms they had suffered for years, could HBOT do the same for people with PTSD?* If true, as that psychiatrist had suggested to me, the potential impact across Israel and beyond could be dramatic.

"Almost everyone in Israel serves in the military. We all know brothers, sisters, or friends who were injured," she said in an interview for this book. "Their trauma from combat events dating back fifty years or more has created one of the biggest wounds for our society. If I could study combat veterans with PTSD, I told Shai, I would change my career to work in the Hyperbarics Institute at Shamir."

"My mission now is to help bring a light into this field. Some veterans I know feel real shame about the condition, that if they just try harder, they will get better. I want to help these guys see that they have a real brain wound, that their symptoms are not imagined. And that they can recover."

Sustaining Gains from HBOT

We didn't know what we should expect to hear later from veterans who participated in the first PTSD study. A follow-up study two years after that first study confirmed HBOT's continuing impact in the lives of most of those patients after they departed the Shamir clinic.[1] Their reports have been uplifting, broadly. Some told their own physicians or Israel's Ministry of Defense physicians that participating in the first PTSD clinical study was life-changing for them.

Most measures of improvements we recorded during the study of reduced symptoms and other improvements continued to hold. Most participants reported they had totally stopped or reduced prescription drugs they had been taking.

Two measures improved over time: cognitive abilities and mood. Those changes may reflect a change in the way people perceive the world. Safety and self-esteem can only be rebuilt after core symptoms are in retreat.

"After their treatments in the hyperbaric chamber, many of them were able to return to work, to get married, to have kids," says Keren. She conducted many of the participant interviews and stays in touch with dozens of veterans we have treated. "Their social performance is much better. The number who are married and holding a job has almost doubled. Some had not left their homes since the Second Lebanon War in 2006; and some not since the Gaza War in 2014."

After analyzing results from the first study, Israel's Ministry of Defense agreed HBOT treatments are effective. The Ministry now covers expenses for HBOT treatments for veterans with PTSD who apply for it. In the first year after that welcomed decision, we treated more than a hundred former combat soldiers with a PTSD diagnosis.

We have kept the Veterans Affairs Department in the United States apprised of our HBOT and PTSD investigations and treatments for Israeli veterans. We hope they make the same commitment to PTSD treatment for U.S. veterans. The current situation is unbearable: the Veterans Health Administration reported in 2016 that 27 percent of soldiers seeking care who served in Iraq, Afghanistan, or both, were diagnosed with PTSD.

The symptoms become worse as these veterans age chronologically. We don't see or hear enough about this in the news, but every hour on average, a U.S. military veteran commits suicide. Many of those veterans from the Iraq and Afghan conflicts are taking huge amounts of psychiatric medications. Prescribing psychiatric medications for PTSD is like giving an opioid for pain. It doesn't address the cause of the medical problem.

We need to treat the biology of this wound in the brain, stimulating neuroplasticity with the output of HBOT—hyperoxic–hypoxic paradox (HHP) and hypoxia-inducible factor (HIF). As our research demonstrated, once that wound recovers, normal brain functions return and symptoms of PTSD recede.

How the Pathology of PTSD Unfolds in the Brain

Our insight is that in PTSD, we have a memory encoding problem. Whenever we have a negative, high-stress experience, a surge of energy in the hippocampus disrupts the brain's ability to encode that memory, to preserve it as a past event. Think of the brain as a machine, or an energy-based mechanism, that anticipates and expects the world to look a certain way. A huge, unexpected event like a traumatic experience creates a break in the appropriate way we should perceive the world.

The autonomic nervous system, which regulates our heart rate, blood pressure, respiration, and sexual arousal, becomes overloaded. The hippocampus that normally connects all parts of a memory doesn't know what to do with this overwhelming traumatic experience. It can't integrate or encode these traumatic memories in the normal way, so the experience is replayed over and over, during the night, as nightmares, or as flashbacks during the day.

To understand the memory gap related to PTSD, there are two types of memories we should be familiar with: *implicit* and *explicit* memories. An *implicit memory* is something our brains register unconsciously initially and then tap into unconsciously. For example, we can perform certain tasks such as riding a bicycle without thinking about, without any conscious awareness of, some prior experience. An *explicit memory* is the conscious, intentional recollection of facts, previous experiences, and concepts. Most of us can easily recall an explicit memory when we want to speak or write about it. The situation could be as simple as what we had for dinner last night.

We all have bad experiences. Those memories can make us sad or anxious, but they are related to a past time and location; an explicit memory. The memory coding problem in PTSD generates a gap between implicit and explicit memories. We relive the past in the present; the implicit is not well connected with explicit. You can easily replay emotions and feelings associated with the traumatic event, but you don't have the explicit memory of the event.

For example, Israeli soldiers who came under fire in Lebanon may not be able to express with words what happened in the months and years after that traumatic event. The event wasn't encoded well in their hippocampus. Yet a sudden spontaneous cue such as a slammed door or some other unexpected loud sound, a smell, or even a taste in their mouths can trigger the same fight-or-flight emotions they experienced during combat in Lebanon. We classify physiological responses triggered by these cues as *intrusive symptoms.*

The body vividly recreates those same feelings and emotions, but there is no conscious recall of the event that planted the original feelings and emotions associated with it.

Again, symptoms of PTSD arise because of this gap between specific memories and sensations retained from that memory. The area of the brain that governs flight-or-fight response, the amygdala, has raced into overdrive reflexively with that burst of energy to help us quickly assess and respond to dangers. It is as though the limbic system is sounding a fire alarm inside the brain that urges you to react . . . but there is no fire.

Meanwhile, the prefrontal cortex is markedly subdued, neurologically. As a result, our ability to manage limbic activities and control our responses to sudden stress weakens. You have these frightening feelings and sensations but cannot connect any experience with these feelings and sensations.

Hearing or seeing fireworks nearby might make your heart beat faster or cause you to gasp for air. You feel as if you are back on a battlefield. You become intensely vigilant, even aggressive.

The hippocampus, which should integrate the memory fractions, withdraws from normal signaling activity. This sustained imbalance in the brain between an amygdala thrust into overdrive and the hippocampus subdued by flickering or absent neuronal activity may be the defining neurology of PTSD.

It is not enough to give medicine to someone to help them relax or sleep better, just as prescribing an opioid to relieve someone's pain does not solve the problem. We need to understand the biological aspects of the pain, then do what is necessary to correct the biological malfunctions.

For PTSD, the core problem is a biologically malfunctioning brain tissue—it is a wound in the brain. As with other brain injuries, that wound needs to be healed; its healthy functioning needs to be restored. In the clinical setting, we know that the wound is recovered when the veteran tells us, "The past has become the past. It is now part of my history, of who I am today, but I am not living it anymore." Once this happens, a patient's PTSD symptoms retreat. The next step, which must be included, is to teach them how to live successfully again in ways that are appropriate to whatever their circumstances are in the modern world.

It is the same approach we have for athletes suffering from a leg fracture. They will collapse if they try to run on a leg with a stress fracture. Once the leg is fully healed, you can train them to compete again in their sports—football, basketball, baseball, running—whatever they are.

Flashbacks, Nightmares, Sudden Sounds

An estimated 7 percent of adults in the U.S. general population experience PTSD during their lifetimes, but as medical researchers have emphasized, "the prevalence among military veterans is much higher."[2]

As many as 20 percent of combat veterans in particular struggle with the many symptoms of PTSD,[3] such as flashbacks to a terrifying event either experienced or witnessed, nightmares, and reacting to sudden sounds with uncontrollable emotional distress. Many veterans also suffer depression and hopelessness. They avoid activities with family, friends, and other social groups—similar to the women in our fibromyalgia studies who were traumatized by childhood sexual abuse.

Psychotherapy treatments designed to ease trauma symptoms, followed by prescription drug therapies when psychotherapy fails, are less effective than once believed. Recent studies show that only up to 40 percent respond to any of the current available treatments.

Authors of a 2015 PTSD study of U.S. military veterans concluded in an update of that study in 2020, "Even when PTSD symptoms improved following treatment, they often persisted to some degree at or above diagnostic thresholds for PTSD, indicating that patients got better but rarely got well."[4] Meanwhile, as people with PTSD grow older, they gradually lose their ability to recognize their condition, their behaviors. Mental deterioration accelerates.

Advanced Imaging for Detecting, Confirming PTSD

Of course, just like a stress fracture in a bone, a wound in the brain cannot be seen from the outside or by standard anatomical imaging. You need metabolic mapping to understand how well the central nervous system is functioning in any given location (metabolic/functional mapping). This is what positron emission tomography (PET) or functional MRI scans do. They illustrate metabolic activity in tissue; with PET and functional MRI scans, we can see the stress fracture. This metabolic/functional brain imaging allows us now to see the "stress wounds" in the brain.

Unfortunately, we do not yet have well-defined biomarkers that enable us to make a PTSD diagnosis. These diagnoses are still based on interviews and questionnaires.

If you are rushed to an emergency room with chest pain, medical staff will quickly conduct tests to determine if you are having a myocardial infarction, a heart attack, or something less urgent, such as a panic attack. You are given a heart enzyme, a biomarker to determine if your heart has been damaged. Heart functions are analyzed by electrocardiograms that measure a heart's electrical activity. These objective measurements help shape diagnosis.

The lack of objective measures for diagnosing PTSD has significant consequences for soldiers beyond medical treatment. Some soldiers will do anything they can to be discharged, especially with some form of compensation. Complaining about having any of the twenty symptoms associated with PTSD is a frequent strategy. Military officials routinely assume that an active-duty soldier or veteran out of the service who is voicing these complaints is lying. Why? Because veterans verified officially as PTSD sufferers receive compensation.

On the other hand, many worthy veterans refuse to apply for therapy and compensation they deserve—and in many cases, they desperately need it. They were elite fighters, the best of the armed forces, but many would rather not run a gauntlet of official suspicion after serving honorably and fighting with valor.

We understood the motivations of these two types of soldiers and veterans; one was to qualify for compensation by lying about symptoms, the other to avoid scornful scrutiny by not reporting legitimate, destructive symptoms. Having a well-defined biomarker would solve both problems. In time, we believe advanced functional MRI and DTI (diffusion tensor tractography) imaging technology will change this. New blood tests also have potential to become PTSD biomarkers.

"As scientists, we know how to measure things," Keren says. "That has not been possible with PTSD because measurements have always been subjective, based on opinions of patients, psychologists, or medical professionals. A diagnosis was based on someone's experience or perception, not science. They have not had tools for objective measurement."

In 2021, we initiated one of the most comprehensive studies to date on veterans suffering from PTSD to identify the biological fingerprint of PTSD. We are evaluating veterans who served together, exposed to the same situations and environment. Some developed PTSD; some did not.

All participants are undergoing a comprehensive analysis that includes functional MRI and DTI data, evaluations of intensive blood tests, the autonomic nervous system, and more. Deep learning and AI technologies are in place to help interpret results from the rigorous evaluations.

We hope the answers will lead us to a biomarker. This is the highly urgent, crucial element that medical professionals—and millions of affected people—need to confirm scientifically and with much higher probability a diagnosis of PTSD.

It is worth repeating here that we hope the same HBOT treatments that have helped hundreds of Israeli military veterans recover from

PTSD—and drawn the Israeli Ministry of Defense's financial support for veterans who seek it—will be made available for the thousands of American military veterans suffering from PTSD and post-concussion syndrome (PCS). The high rate of suicide among military veterans burdened with PTSD is a tragedy, a major health crisis. The situation is urgent.

Key Takeaways

1. Many veterans with PTSD suffer depression and hopelessness in addition to flashbacks and nightmares, and they often react to sudden sounds with uncontrollable emotional distress.
2. PTSD is a real brain wound, a biological event, not solely psychological and not an indicator of a character flaw.
3. HBOT helps reduce PTSD symptoms by rebuilding damaged brain tissue and restoring healthy neuron functioning.
4. Based on our research, Israel's Ministry of Defense now covers HBOT treatment expenses for veterans with PTSD after we complete an evaluation and find that these veterans are suitable for HBOT.

CHAPTER 9

Long COVID: Mysteries, Discoveries, and Cures

It was December 2019 when reports of a lethal virus of unknown origins—and no known cures—first surfaced in Wuhan, the sprawling capital city of eleven million people in China's Hubei province.

We in the global medical and science community were caught flat-footed. *What are we facing? How does the virus spread? How can we diagnose and treat it? What medicines might boost our immune systems for defense against it? If you recover from one infection, will antibodies protect against a second? If so, for how long?*

Lacking answers, with hospitals overwhelmed with dying and seriously ill patients, countries across the globe shut their borders to foreigners. Civilians were ordered into lockdown, crippling economies and paralyzing essential social networks in education, religion, and entertainment. At what costs? For how long? Desperate for answers, governments turned to public health officials, physicians, and medical researchers.

Like many in Israel's medical professions, my clinical and research teams and I were quick to respond. While doing everything within our power to treat the streams of patients with respiratory distress surging into emergency rooms and pandemic wards, we needed answers, too.

To search for them, we worked late hours in Shamir Medical Center labs. Physicians needed new diagnostic measures to detect the virus. They needed solid biological insights about immune responses to the virus. This is where we focused our energies.

We, of course, were not lone actors. Scientists had a common enemy in the pandemic larger than individual egos. Everyone was sharing research. Zoom calls were happening at all hours. Insightful data that scientists habitually had kept to themselves until they published were freely shared in pre-publication tweets, blogs, and articles online. This was an unprecedented historical passage in science for accelerating discovery, a point we'll revisit later in this chapter.

Our team explored how the immune system responded to infections of this new coronavirus, SARS-CoV-2. We analyzed how long people retain antibodies that fight the infection and identified tools to best measure the presence of those antibodies.

As we followed up with patients a year after their acute infections, we started noticing unexpected long-term effects. Roughly one of every five patients complained about cognitive decline, brain fog, and fatigue, but we could not find any correlation between these long-term disabilities and the severity of an initial infection and age of a patient.

We wondered, *What is going on? What are we dealing with?*

To establish facts and construct answers, we had to initiate a rigorous study. Many colleagues in the medical professions were dismissing these ongoing symptoms as unsurprising psychological reactions to pandemic stress, but with our deepening knowledge of the biochemistry in brain injuries and neurological disorders, we were thinking differently.

By January 2022, more than 300 million cases of infections globally had been confirmed. Most of these patients would recover, but the World Health Organization estimated that between 10 and 30 percent—thirty to ninety million people—would go on to experience persistent symptoms three months and on after the COVID-19 infection, with devastating impacts on their quality of life.[1,2] A month later, in February, an estimated sixteen million adults in the United States alone had been affected by these post-COVID symptoms, with perhaps two million to four million lost to the workforce.[3]

Investigating an Expansive Biological Breakdown

The clock for what soon became known as a Long COVID diagnosis starts if symptoms have persisted for more than two months after infection, and those systems cannot be explained by a different diagnosis.[4] More than twenty symptoms have been codified. They can span from physical problems such as extreme fatigue and insomnia, brain fog characterized by a slower pace of thinking (neurocognitive) and memory loss, and loss of taste and smell, to psychiatric issues such as depression, anxiety, and PTSD. Multiple organ systems can be damaged. Given this wide expanse of biological distress, we can regard Long COVID more as an umbrella diagnosis covering multiple symptoms.

By early 2024, medical scientists had not yet determined the specific metabolic breakdowns—the specific pathologies—that cause Long COVID, but we had learned much more since the pandemic first appeared.

We knew by 2022 that the virus can damage the brain in various ways. We also knew that treatment options studied for Long COVID, such as special diets, psychotherapy sessions, and anti-inflammation medications, had proved disappointing. Alarmingly, patients in otherwise good health with mild initial infections from the virus could develop Long COVID symptoms. Vaccinations help reduce the risk for Long COVID effects, but they do not eliminate them.

Frontal Lobe, Bloodstream Infections

Long COVID appears to be a neurological brain disorder. The virus can penetrate the brain directly through the bone just above our nose, the cribriform plate, or through the bloodstream. A direct penetration mostly involves the frontal lobe, which plays a critical role in many cognitive and behavioral functions that make us uniquely human. It is the largest and most complex of the brain's lobes.

Here are some of the frontal lobe's key functions.

- **Executive Function:** Helps us plan, make decisions, and carry out complex tasks. It also plays a role in working memory, which allows us to hold information in our minds while we manipulate it.
- **Social Behavior:** Helps us understand and respond appropriately to social cues and plays a role in self-awareness by regulating our emotions and social behavior.
- **Attention and Concentration:** Helps us focus our attention and maintain concentration on tasks, especially those that require sustained effort.
- **Language:** While many areas of the brain participate in how we process language, the frontal lobe's key role in this complex task is how we produce language, such as generating speech and articulating words.
- **Problem-solving:** Helps us analyze complex problems and develop solutions, using both logical and creative thinking.

The virus may also enter the brain through the bloodstream, where endothelial cells form an inner lining of the vessels. The virus can bind the ACE-2 receptor (angiotensin converting enzyme-2), which is expressed naturally by endothelial cells. That binding of the ACE-2 receptor can create havoc: activating the clotting system when the bloodstream has no need for clots. Neuronal and glial cells can also express ACE-2 receptors.

When the spike protein of a SARS-CoV-2 virus attaches to ACE-2, the clotting system goes awry. Small blood clots form. They can damage the lungs, heart, and brain. We saw in patients how a young person's brain can age dramatically as clotting creates blockages in blood vessels and, often, a series of minor strokes as clots travel into the brain.

Given what we had demonstrated about HBOT's effectiveness in nonhealing brain wounds from other neurological brain disorders—stroke, concussion, fibromyalgia, and PTSD—we asked, *Is it likely that HBOT also can heal brain damage and quiet the myriad symptoms from Long COVID?*

Once More: HBOT, Neuroplasticity, and Healing

For our first clinical study of HBOT and patients with Long COVID, we recruited seventy-three patients who were paced at random into an HBOT treatment group or a placebo/sham group. Participants were at least eighteen years old, with cognitive decline and other symptoms harming their quality of life lasting for at least three months following a test that confirmed their COVID-19 infection.

In addition to cognitive functions, we evaluated other mental symptoms, quality of sleep, pain disturbance, and cardiac functions. High-resolution brain perfusion scans with MRI-DTI (magnetic resonance imaging and diffusion tensor tractography) and functional MRI were part of baseline and post-treatment/placebo evaluations. *Nature-Scientific Reports* published the first scientific article with results on our study in July 2022.[5]

We chose a shorter, forty-day treatment protocol of HBOT sessions for this study rather than the usual sixty sessions we had established to safely induce brain neuroplasticity. Why? We anticipated patients might have a significant, spontaneous recovery during any period of time they were in HBOT protocols or the placebo/sham group. A shorter treatment period could still demonstrate recovery from Long COVID symptoms, we reasoned, which was all we needed to show the efficacy of HBOT treatments.

In fact, people in the placebo group showed little if any effects from spontaneous recovery that might have eased the severity of their symptoms. Our post-evaluation review suggested that patients adjusted to their limitations because objective measures of multiple symptoms did not improve.

Put another way, patients in the placebo group became used to their new limitations. They become used to being less productive. They understood less of what they were able to read. They needed to rest more during the day and adjusted to deepening memory loss by writing more things down. Their reduced cognitive and physical capabilities became normalized. These were signs of chronic unremitting brain injury.

In contrast, patients who received HBOT with the HHP response had significant biological improvements. We could see in MRI scans the cerebral brain blood flows in gray matter and perfusion across the frontal lobe. As we mentioned earlier, the frontal lobe is where the brain manages attention and short-term memory. Cognitive functions improved significantly along with improving brain biology that we tracked in brain scans.

The treatment group's mental or psychiatric symptoms retreated in ways similar to what we had observed in HBOT studies with PTSD patients. Participants in the treatment group had less anxiety and depression. Moreover, as we observed in our fibromyalgia studies years before, generalized pain symptoms in the HBOT-treated group also dissolved.

Fatigue, more specifically mental fatigue, is one of the most common symptoms reported by post-COVID patients; in our study, 77 percent of participants cited fatigue as a major distressing factor in their struggles to recover from the original virus infection. Many post-COVID clients in our clinics struggle to read more than five minutes at a time.

Chronic fatigue syndrome and post-COVID diagnosis share many overlapping symptoms. They include fatigue, pain, reduced daily activity, depression, and other psychiatric disorders, and a worsening of symptoms generally after even minor physical or mental exertion.

One of the important things we gained from the Long COVID study was additional insight on the biology of PTSD. Young people with Long COVID who were otherwise healthy, who did not have any severe acute COVID disease, and who were not exposed to any emotional traumatic event suddenly started to suffer PTSD-like symptoms. Their functional brain damage caused by a tiny virus was strongly correlated with what most physicians diagnosed as psychiatric disorders.

This gave us new insights into the biology of those symptoms. We could track with functional MRI protocols how recovery developed as oxygen perfusion during the HBOT treatments improved in the amygdala and insula networks. Later, we could match patients' improved scores on post-treatment psychiatric assessments with the healthier structure of their amygdala circuits. The hyperoxic–hypoxic paradox had induced regeneration in both functional connectivity and micro-structural parameters of the amygdala circuit. The amygdala circuit is where our brains manage the fight-or-flight response.

This biochemical healing closely matched improvements in psychiatric symptoms associated with Long COVID. What if the same regenerative steps with HHP through HBOT could also cure other psychiatric disorders still widely regarded as incurable?

Today, we know Long COVID could be a trigger for central sensitization syndromes such as fibromyalgia—and the same symptoms of generalized pain in the body plus others for which there appear to be no direct medical cause (somatization). As we demonstrated in our previous fibromyalgia studies, once damage in those brain regions was repaired, the pain dissolved, and patients were able to live more normal lives.

The concept of reverse engineering applies here. If brain scans show damage in areas responsible for pain signal interpretations, we can anticipate symptoms of fibromyalgia. If we see damage in areas responsible for anxiety control or symptoms related to PTSD, we can anticipate clinical presentation of PTSD. If there is damage in mood-related brain regions, we can anticipate depression.

This and different Long COVID studies by others added more support to our findings that HHP can induce neuroplasticity and improve brain functions even months to years after an acute injury.

To reiterate once more, our HBOT protocol for fluctuating pressure and oxygen concentration in the chamber generates the HHP. This biochemical cascade triggers three core metabolic benefits: (1) a surge in the proliferation and migration of stem cells; (2) restoration of a better, more normal metabolism in cells by improving mitochondria's role in transporting and converting oxygen to energy in molecules; and (3) increased perfusion as more new blood vessels are being generated.

From Dispiriting Siege to Again Running up Mountain Trails

Patrick* was a remarkably fit outdoorsman and athlete—sailing on oceans, running in mountains—and a global shipping executive. Then early in 2021, an intense bout with COVID-19 and severe dehydration landed the fifty-five-year-old Dutchman in an intensive care ward for three weeks.

Within days, tiny air sacs in his lungs filled with fluid leaking from blood vessels.[6] He had contracted a type of lung inflammation we call *pneumonitis* (pneumonia, an infection, is a form of pneumonitis). Breathing was so difficult that he required high-flow oxygen treatments for a week before he was stable enough to go home. "I could barely walk," he recalls. "It was a big blow. I had been on top of my game."

A week after returning home, his expectations for recovery collapsed.

A painful blood clot blocked an artery in one of his lungs; a cure required anti-coagulation medication. Attempts to resume regular exercise routines failed as his breathing quickly became labored. Brain fog and memory loss sewed confusion and frustration in his work. "I was in worse shape than I had thought." He was back in the ICU.

Patrick was under siege from multiple symptoms of what at the time we were labeling as "post-COVID." When we first evaluated him at our clinic in Dubai, we speculated that those symptoms might reflect two key aspects of brain injury we had seen in patients treated in our prior HBOT studies on stroke, concussion, fibromyalgia, etc. One was a lack of brain oxygen related to narrowed or blocked blood flows and weakened blood vessels damaged by the virus; the other an uncontrolled response by the inflammation system that can damage healthy neuronal tissue. Both can be

* At Patrick's request, we are not disclosing his surname.

responsible for chronic, unremitting decline in the brain functions of Long COVID patients.

MRI scans confirmed metabolic dysfunction of tissue in areas of Patrick's brain that manage multitask thinking, memory, and more. For treatment, we designed a full three-month HBOT program (sixty sessions: two hours daily, five days each week) from mid April to mid July. We supported these "dives" in the hyperbaric chamber with programs to sharpen his diet and restore his physical fitness and to administer brain scans to track and interpret ongoing neurological changes.

"I can never remember ever being treated by so many doctors, looking at all components of my body, from head to toe. I embraced all this as much as I could, all for a survival perspective. I wanted to keep my job, to keep on living, to keep being an outdoors person and be there for my family."

After five sessions, his breathing began to improve and muscle aches after exercise faded. By fifteen sessions, he noted less fatigue and rising levels of energy. "You feel unstoppable." After twenty sessions (roughly one month), he was hiking again and doing extreme trail runs in the mountains. All with the same breathing and exercise capacity he enjoyed before the COVID-19 infection. His memory and multitasking abilities reclaimed pre-COVID-19 levels as well.

Two months later, after the sixty sessions, Patrick's physical and mental scores had risen much higher. His maximum oxygen consumption during exercise (VO_2 Max) improved 34 percent. His capacity to exhale rapidly and forcefully (FVC) jumped 44 percent, and his maximal working metabolic rate (METS) rose 34 percent. And, in one impressive indication that his biological aging course had been reversed, telomere lengths on his chromosomes increased 46 percent.

"Basically, I got regenerated and became *younger* in my fifty-six-year-old body," Patrick says. "I was very fortunate. I've met many Long COVID patients who were struggling after nine months and still could not walk up stairs. I was running up mountains."

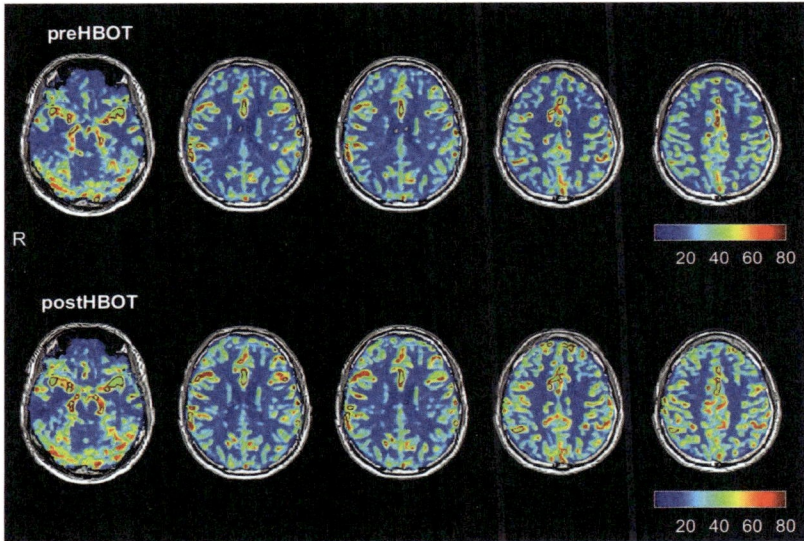

Figure 9-1: Brain perfusion magnetic resonance imaging before and after Patrick's hyperbaric oxygen therapy. The upper row represents brain perfusion three months after the acute infection, before hyperbaric oxygen therapy. The lower row shows the perfusion magnetic resonance imaging after completing the hyperbaric oxygen therapy protocol.

Mapping the Brain's Neurological Breakdowns

Many Long COVID symptoms originate in the brain's frontal lobe. Neurological control rooms there are responsible for maintaining healthy functions for attention, short-term memory, and psychological moods. Studies showed that the inhaled COVID-19 virus can penetrate this region through tissue behind the nasal cavity, a small section of the forward-facing skull known as the cribriform plate.

Once into the brain, the virus can inject its genetic material into neurons and damage them as well as glial cells that help protect and cleanse neuronal networks by, among other things, digesting dead neurons. Studies in the United Kingdom conducted in 2021 and 2022 showed tissue damage especially in gray matter linked to how we sense and filter odors (the olfactory system), and in areas associated with Long COVID setbacks such as brain fog, fatigue, depression, psychological distress, and PTSD.[7]

We took advantage of neurological mapping data accumulated in our first Long COVID study to look in a second study at how HHP promotes improvements in neural pathways, or neuroplasticity, in these patients. We found that the treatments improved the vibrancy and functioning of neural networks that govern emotions.[8]

The biology is clear now, but in the first year after the lockdown, many medical professionals dismissed symptoms we observed as a psychiatric response to social isolation, anxiety, and economic disruptions. We were seeing young, otherwise healthy patients who became anxious or depressed. It was challenging to find specialists to treat them. "It's only mental," they told us.

Elite Athletes, Long COVID, and Career-Threatening Heart Trouble

Our estimate from what we have learned by working with hundreds of elite athletes directly in our clinics and researching the biology of elite performance is that approximately 3 percent of professional athletes had retired prematurely by the end of 2022 because of Long COVID. They no longer could compete at the same level. Whatever treatments they had sought for Long COVID could not help them regain their exceptional mental quickness and physical prowess.

As we noted in chapter 2, many athletes come to our clinics from across the world. Most, like Alon Day, the reigning European NASCAR racing champion at age thirty-one, are highly motivated to improve performance and, often, extend their careers into and beyond their mid-thirties. As we focused intensely on pandemic research, we began seeing more athletes of many ages with Long COVID symptoms, but not a Long COVID diagnosis. They came to us startled and anxious about how rapidly their energy flagged during intense workouts and competitions. *What is wrong?* they wondered.

We learned from studies published by other scientists after Long COVID was codified that patients in the broader population can suffer a range of heart and brain problems. They include reduced blood flows, ruptured blood vessels, blood clots, blocked arteries, sharp chest pains, and abnormal or irregular heartbeats.

Standard echocardiograph tests often indicate that the heart functions of many Long COVID patients are within the "normal range" of synchronous contractions. Their hearts are considered healthy. Yet higher resolution imaging can often identify problems hiding in these contractions. These abnormalities become a bigger concern for anyone, and especially competitive athletes, as demands for peak cardiac performance rise during intensive training exercise or competitions.

We evaluate cardiac functioning as part of our research with all post-COVID patients. Many athletes indeed had those abnormalities. The smooth synchronization of their heart contractions was disrupted; at times, they were too fast, at times too slow. Then, too, abnormal heartbeats might indicate a damaged neuronal autonomic system. Could HBOT correct this? Yes.

We found in a year-long study completed in December 2021 that HBOT improved outcomes on one excellent measure of how well a patient's heart contraction is synchronized.[9] Known as *global longitudinal strain* (GLS), the measure assesses how heart fibers most prone to ischemia or wall damage are functioning. (A subgroup of post-COVID patients who did not receive HBOT had abnormal GLS scores in the cardiac evaluation.)

The anticipated surge in stem cell production and proliferation, rapid replication of oxygen-bearing mitochondria cells, and more abundant circulatory pathways helped them improve.

To the best of our knowledge, this was the first study investigating HBOT on heart functions in Long COVID patients. Moreover, it was the first randomized, placebo control study to prove that HBOT treatments can improve cardiac functions in those patients.

Accelerating the Pace of Discovery

The magnitude of the COVID-19 pandemic has been a tragedy for hundreds of millions of people who died or were severely impaired from the infection. It has slowed or reversed decades of progress in improving healthcare, increasing lifespan, and reducing global poverty, and it piled massive unanticipated debt burdens on governments across the global economy.

Yet, the unprecedented collaboration by medical scientists and health system professionals in response to the pandemic has given us stunning insights into the microbiology and cause of diseases we had struggled to understand. Scientists and medical teams dedicated to solving the mystery shared data in real time. They focused on the global urgency and benefits discoveries could deliver and not on their personal careers.

In almost no time, new vaccine technology and antiviral medications were developed and approved for use. Governments understood that the resilience of society depended on the quality of the medical care they provided for their citizens. Deploying nuclear submarines or lightning-fast stealth fighter jets could not compensate for lack of good medical care.

Understanding more deeply the science of how a virus triggers a neurological problem and how that problem can be corrected is a major, ongoing objective. Studying unmarked symptoms of relatively healthy young persons with COVID-19 infections or post-COVID symptoms led to many insights that we could not have made as quickly and clearly with the standard mice or rat studies. As we homed in on these problems and sought cures for them, we learned more about molecular mishaps in the brain's neural networks related to those symptoms. Put simply, our post-COVID studies opened a window into which parts of the brain correspond with which of the many Long COVID symptoms.

To cite just one example, today we know that the Epstein-Barr virus is a major cause of multiple sclerosis, a degenerative disease of the central nervous system that affects 2.8 million people worldwide. Previously, Epstein-Barr was considered idiopathic, a disease with unknown origins. Physicians have not recommended vaccination for Epstein-Barr because in most cases, the natural immune response clears or contains the infection, a characteristic of what we call self-limiting disease. Now that Epstein-Barr's link to multiple sclerosis has been demonstrated, should we change our thinking?

We all know that the conditions for most of the world's eight billion people today would have been vastly better without the pain and suffering the COVID-19 pandemic caused.

Yet, there is no bad without good. Thousands of Long COVID patients have been treated at our clinics since our first clinical study demonstrating HBOT's efficacy was published in July 2022. The insights we gained from treating and monitoring each young person in our clinics would not have been possible otherwise.

Key Takeaways

1. Long COVID patients who received HBOT had significant benefits in the structure and function of their brains. Cognitive functions improved significantly along

with the improving brain structure and functions tracked in brain scans. HBOT also improved the vibrancy and functioning of neural networks that govern emotions.

2. Long COVID patients who suffer long-term damage in the synchronization of heart contractions can also improve with HBOT. The synchronization damage is related to a decline in exercise performance.

3. Long COVID could be a trigger for central sensitization syndromes such as fibromyalgia—with the same symptoms of generalized pain in the body plus fatigue, brain fog, sleep disturbances, and other generalized symptoms.

4. Once damage in those brain regions is repaired, symptoms dissolve, the quality of life improves, and patients are able to live more normal lives.

CHAPTER 10

Alzheimer's Disease

We have seen to this point in Part II how the research, clinical studies, and patients' personal stories of recovery following HBOT treatments improve conditions related to five distinct brain injuries: stroke, concussion, fibromyalgia, PTSD, and Long COVID.

And you know by now that abnormally low cerebral blood flow, ischemia, is at the root of them all. People ask me all the time: "Might this be true as well for Alzheimer's disease? Could a malfunction in tissue biology that causes ischemia and lack of oxygen in the brain play a crucial role in the failing health and behavior of people who develop Alzheimer's disease?"

We began looking into those questions shortly after finishing the HBOT stroke and concussion studies. According to the Alzheimer's Association, an estimated 6.7 million Americans in the fast-growing cohort of people aged sixty-five or older suffered from this fatal disease in 2023.[1] Total healthcare costs to treat them exceeded $300 billion and are projected to rise beyond $1 trillion by 2050.[2]

In recent years, we have been among dozens of investigators hoping to push the boundaries of what we know about preventing and treating Alzheimer's. Much work remains, but we are optimistic.

We need to be meticulous here about what we know, what we don't know, and what might be discovered in the next few years, so we'll lean more in this chapter on the science in Alzheimer's disease research drawn from physiology, biology, and medicine. Many terms we have already introduced. We won't include any patient examples or stories because we have not completed any Alzheimer's clinical studies. Let's begin.

Beta-Amyloid Is Present but Not the Primary Cause of Alzheimer's

In the past, most physicians and medical scientists believed or were taught that an abnormal amyloid protein known as *beta-amyloid* is the primary cause of Alzheimer's. Yet recent studies show that while beta-amyloid is indeed present as Alzheimer's develops, **it is not the primary cause of Alzheimer's.** That insight is the most important takeaway in this chapter.

Under normal, healthy physiological conditions, amyloid proteins help cells and tissues maintain their chemical structure. But misshapen chemical structures of amyloid proteins can be destructive and often are. The presence of malformed amyloid proteins is one of the criteria physicians cite when diagnosing Alzheimer's. Recent studies have also suggested a potential connection between amyloid and other neurodegenerative maladies such as Parkinson's disease.

We can think of beta-amyloid as a biomarker for a patient who may be at risk of developing full Alzheimer's in the same way that an electrocardiogram (which records a heart's rhythm and electrical activity) or enzymes of myocardium (cardiac muscle) serve as biomarkers of heart disease caused by ischemia. Neither the electro-cardiogram nor the presence of myocardium enzymes are the primary cause of heart disease.

A 2016 study by Jack C. de la Torre estimated that damage to small blood vessels and reduced blood flows are responsible for the accumulation of the amyloid protein in up to 90 percent of people with Alzheimer's disease.[3]

An earlier study, by N.R. Sims and M.F. Anderson in 2002[4] and another later by J.L. Yang, S. Mukda, and S.D. Chen in 2018[5] showed that when mitochondria are deprived of oxygen, they generate more cell-damaging molecules of reactive oxygen species (ROS) per neuronal cells and fewer new mitochondria.

These and other damaging consequences cause more amyloid to leak from blood vessels and amyloid plaque to build up in blood vessels in the brain. The cascade of breakdowns leads to plaque accumulation that can damage blood flows. When positron emission tomography (PET) scans detect amyloid plaque in a brain with abnormal blood flows, this indicates the presence of Alzheimer's. The most common forms of Alzheimer's develop as people age past sixty-five.[6]

Symptoms begin most commonly with deteriorating short-term memory that worsens and extends to declines in other cognitive skills as amyloid accumulates in cerebral blood vessels. The volume of deteriorating and dead neurons becomes more pronounced in an Alzheimer's brain as the disease progresses and tissue is destroyed.[7]

Medical scientists have calibrated ischemia's relationship to Alzheimer's over time. One key finding is that insufficient blood flows in the brain accelerate the onset of dementia by ten years. About 10 percent of people with dementia develop this condition soon after they suffer an initial stroke. After a second stroke, dementia symptoms rise to more than 40 percent. Within twenty-five years after a stroke, dementia develops in nearly half the cases, an estimated 48 percent.

I want to underscore here that the presence of amyloid in the brain is *not sufficient on its own* to predict with certainty that a patient eventually will develop Alzheimer's disease. Additional factors need to be included in assessing this risk, such as age, genetics, cognitive performance, and the presence of other biomarkers.

Put another way, while the presence of amyloid proteins in people who have not yet displayed any symptoms of Alzheimer's disease may increase their risk of developing the disorder, the prediction rate is influenced by various factors. We need more research to give us a clearer understanding of how frequently the presence of amyloid proteins will develop into Alzheimer's disease. (This calculation is termed the *conversion rate*.)

As the de la Torre analysis showed, as many as 90 percent of people with Alzheimer's exhibit two medical issues: deficient blood flows (cerebral hypoperfusion) and a buildup of amyloid proteins in the walls of blood vessels (amyloid angiopathy).

We might be able to slow or reverse the natural progression of dementia and Alzheimer's if we can intervene sooner to prevent narrowing blood flows in the brain. This is why physicians need to act as early as possible after signs of ischemia have been detected in the brain.

The Many Origins of Ischemia

Damage from vascular pathology, or reduced blood flows, can originate in five ways: atherosclerosis, arteriosclerosis, acute blockages in a vessel that are known as *infarcts* or *strokes*, white matter lesions, and microbleeds.

These cause hypoperfusion, tissue ischemia, chronic inflammation, accelerating deaths of neurons, gliosis or inflammation of glia cells, and cerebral atrophy, or the loss of brain tissue. Moreover, the accumulation of beta-amyloid and tau proteins in vessels becomes more toxic after they combine chemically with phosphoric acid or a phosphate group, a process known as *phosphorylation.*

Other factors that can deposit plaques of fatty material along the inner walls of veins and produce atherosclerosis include hypertension; diabetes mellitus, or abnormally high levels of glucose, or sugar, and abnormally high levels of insulin in the blood; dyslipidemia, or unhealthy levels of fats or lipids in the blood; and obesity.

Need we add what is now widely accepted and often noted? A sedentary lifestyle increases the odds that someone will suffer a serious blood disease—a vascular pathology.

The resulting plethora of chronic ailments from vascular pathology deprives mitochondria of oxygen. This makes mitochondria less efficient in carrying oxygen and converting that oxygen to energy. And there are fewer of them because fewer mitochondria survive to nourish neurons.

Whatever the cause, ischemia makes the blood–brain barrier less effective in preventing toxic material such as bacteria and viruses from entering the brain. That is its main function. Circulating blood is more prone to deliver harmful agents to the brain, namely soluble beta-amyloid, a toxin that contributes to amyloidosis, which is a buildup of protein fragments and plaque that if unchecked can develop into cerebral amyloid angiopathy. Blood vessels damaged by cerebral amyloid angiopathy are more likely to hemorrhage and cause stroke. And, as we noted, origins of dementia and Alzheimer's often are linked to stroke.

Breakdowns in the molecular integrity of arteries and tiny vessels and the buildup of protein fragments in the brain are common signs of advancing Alzheimer's disease. We can detect these specific warnings on MRI sequences displaying conditions of tissue deep inside the brain: more tissue wearing away (rapidly intensifying white matter), small hemorrhages or microbleeds, and small buildups of fluids, or lacunes.

Genetics matter as well. Carriers of the ε4 allele of the apolipo-
protein E (APOE) gene do not efficiently break down beta-amyloid
plaques. This mutation makes the healthy functioning of lipid transport, synaptic integrity, glucose metabolism, and blood flows in the
brain more prone to mishaps. Cases classified as early onset Alzheimer's occurring before age fifty-five often are caused by some specific
gene mutation.

Neuro-Inflammation and Ischemia

Peak performance in any region of the brain depends on healthy cerebral blood flows. These healthy flows will shift naturally to an area of
the brain that is more active in a given moment, because it is being
charged with some immediate task.

Think of Alon Day's visual processing speed receiving surging blood
flows during a NASCAR race as opposed to another less active area of
his brain, perhaps one for recalling a calculus equation or a childhood
memory. His peak performance, as with anyone, depends on brain
molecules reaching the upper limits of oxygen consumption.

What happens, conversely, with declining capacity of oxygen
consumption? Restricted blood flows induce tissue ischemia and
hypoxia, which ignite a massive response from the brain's innate
immune system. If the damaged blood flow is not corrected quickly,
this innate immune system will continue to respond so intensively
that neurons and glia cells will be damaged. This chronic condition
may cause nerve cells in the brain gradually to lose function and
eventually die.

How? A damaging physiological cascade occurs during
neuro-inflammation that escalates the loss of neurons, disrupts the
neuronal network permanently, and further accelerates the destructive
inflammatory cycle.

Glia and astrocyte cells are activated as early as a few minutes after an ischemic event such as a stroke. They belong to the central nervous system's first line of defense, the immune system's immediate response, and trigger a wider response for other immune cells to come and "take part in the party." A rush of inflammation follows.

The number of tiny defense cells, or neutrophils, produced following ischemia directly corresponds to the size of the ischemic brain injury. These small white blood cells, as well as T and B lymphocytes, natural killer cells, mast cells, and dendritic cells, infiltrate the brain and concentrate around regions where blood flows and oxygen supplies have been restricted. At a later stage, larger white blood cells, or macrophages, become more dominant. Macrophages' role is to eat bacteria and other foreign invaders if any appear; yet in cases of neuro-inflammation triggered by ischemia and hypoxia, these invaders are not present.

Accumulation of Beta-Amyloid and Phosphorylated Tau

Amyloid protein is a neurotoxic substance that induces intracellular processes in post-ischemic neurons, astrocytes, and microglia; this further enhances injury and death of neuronal and glial cells after ischemia occurs. Beta-amyloid is a peptide with a chain of thirty-eight to forty-three amino acids. The sequential breaking of the bonds between amino acids and proteins of amyloid precursor protein (APP) generates these long peptide chains by producing fragments known as *beta-* and *gamma-secretases*.

Though the exact physiological function of APP has not been identified, the overproduction of beta-amyloid generated from this substance disturbs normal activity of the nervous system. The beta-amyloid is widely known to be present as Alzheimer's disease develops. APP also has been identified as a factor contributing to emerging Alzheimer's when beta-amyloid is not cleared or degraded by the immune response.

Following stroke or some other ischemia, beta-amyloid plaques can be seen in several regions of the brain: hippocampus, thalamus, brain cortex, corpus callosum, and around lateral ventricles.* In response to damage of the brain–blood barrier, the influx of inflammatory cytokines, together with the soluble form of beta-amyloid, is increased. (Cytokines are small proteins that allow cells to communicate.) A burst of cytokines released by the immune system accelerates the damaging pathophysiological cascade that can develop into Alzheimer's.

The other hallmark of Alzheimer's disease, the tau protein, accumulates following diminished blood flows in cells with special roles in the central nervous system—microglia, astrocytes, and oligodendrocytes, as well as in the hippocampus and brain cortex.

Hyperphosphorylation of tau, a signaling mechanism that cells use to regulate how they reproduce, dominates in neuronal cells and can lead to troubles in cell growth or development. This bad actor in those circumstances is present under normal metabolism as neurons die off. Tau protein has also been detected in human plasma samples after brain injuries caused by diminished blood flows, and it correlates with the progression of neuronal damage after an event such as stroke caused by diminished blood flows.

---

* APP cleavage via beta- and gamma-secretase to form beta-amyloid is known as the *amyloidogenic pathway*.

Karin Elman-Shina:
Prevention to Avoid Alzheimer's

Dr. Karin Elman-Shina is a specialist in neurology and cognitive disorders. Early in her medical career, she was an investigator in trials of several medications and therapies aimed at preventing Alzheimer's, mild cognitive impairment, and even attention deficit hyperactivity disorder (ADHD). None, unfortunately, proved effective.[8]

In recent years, Karin has been keen to show her patients how improving nutrition, sleep, and physical exercise, and lowering stress (among other steps) can reduce the risk of Alzheimer's. "I went back to the roots of medicine, to biochemistry, focusing as a physician on how disease happens and to intervene as early as possible," she says. She has contributed to several scientific papers, including in 2022 as my co-author for the *Frontiers in Aging Neuroscience* article, "Ischemia as a common trigger for Alzheimer's disease."[9]

In the passage that follows, Karin describes some of her current ideas about the science and preventive health steps for taking on Alzheimer's.

People with diabetes have a major risk of developing cognitive decline associated with Alzheimer's. We see people who follow the standard Western diet despite being aware of an alarming rise in glucose levels in their blood. Many of them expect that prescription medications will reduce those glucose levels and reverse the expected damage, but it doesn't work like that.

If we listen to our bodies, check ourselves occasionally, and pay attention to preventive measures, we have better chances of preventing or delaying cognitive decline. The main goal is prevention, to not have to deal at all with that increase in blood glucose or any other factor that leads to increased risk of Alzheimer's.

A healthy diet, regular exercise, and fasting are all good elements for prevention. In many cases, patients who change their diet can reduce their blood glucose to healthy levels and even eliminate the need for medications.

We have various treatment options today apart from the few medications that can be prescribed. For patients with ischemia of the brain, HBOT might be very helpful in improving blood flows, oxygenation, reducing inflammation, and inducing regeneration. However, in some cases it won't be enough. That is why I put a major emphasis on other interventions such as ketogenic or low-carb nutrition, improving sleep, fasting, and cognitive and physical exercise. I rarely prescribe medications.

Visualizing very small areas of the brain has been a game-changer for us in the last decade or so. We can see if the total brain or a specific part is shrinking. We can identify conditions that may lead to cognitive decline. For example, as people age, blood vessels tend to constrict. This can lead to minor strokes that may later cause patients to develop cognitive decline and Alzheimer's.

Testing for Alzheimer's enables us to better understand what is going on and treat root causes instead of just symptoms. Different imaging modalities such as MRI show the brain's anatomy, PET scans show how certain brain tissues function, and lab tests show nutritional deficiencies, inflammatory states, and other factors that physicians need to address.

The main point is that we have more effective options now to improve the cognition and quality of life for a patient diagnosed with mild cognitive impairment.

As Dr. Elman-Shina's early professional experiences suggest, many clinical drug trials targeting beta-amyloid and tau proteins in various forms have failed to improve cognitive skills. The failure of the drugs in these studies to improve thinking skills suggests that these proteins are not the main drivers of Alzheimer's. To be sure, some trials did show a welcomed weakening and clearance of beta-amyloid and tau proteins.

Alzheimer's has been described as having multiple causes. These include genetic and environmental factors, age-related events, and pathological conditions such as diabetes, traumatic brain injury (TBI), and imbalances or variations in gut microbiota that make us more vulnerable to intestinal disease. Each of these affects how beta-amyloid forms and is collected.

White matter lesions and microhemorrhages, dyslipidemia, altered brain insulin signaling, and insulin resistance all contribute to tau and beta-amyloid pathogenesis. Moreover, we can see the biochemical links between the pathophysiology of Alzheimer's and ischemia by observing three changes: damage to mitochondria, hypoperfusion, and inflammation (immune system).

Each of these three has become a new target for developing pharmaceuticals to treat Alzheimer's.

Interventions to Reverse Brain Ischemia and Improve Metabolism

The brains of healthy aging adults naturally experience some shrinking, but most of the tens of billions of neurons inside our craniums remain active.

Once Alzheimer's has reached the full or late stage, the volume of brain tissue has shrunk dramatically. This is the main reason why HBOT or any other therapeutic intervention has no significant potential effect on reversing late-stage dementia and Alzheimer's. HBOT requires brain tissue, but at this late stage the tissue has lost its capacity to function normally to rebuild viable active neurons and potent blood vessels. Yet during the earlier stage of mild cognitive impairment there is much we can do to delay or even reverse symptoms of cognitive decline.

One sweeping study involving more than 2,000 participants at risk for developing Alzheimer's in several countries, including the United States, is especially encouraging. This two-year, randomized-control trial completed in 2015 demonstrated that positive changes in diet and exercise, as well as social stimulation and routine drills to bolster intellectual skills, did indeed maintain and improve brain health. More to the point, collectively they prevented the onset of dementia. This is widely known as the FINGER trial, the acronym for Finnish Geriatric Intervention Study to Prevent Cognitive Impairment and Disability.[10]

Each cardiovascular risk factor examined in the study had been identified previously as contributing to dementia diagnoses. These included hypertension, smoking, obesity, high levels in the blood of lipids such as cholesterol and triglycerides (hyperlipidemia), diabetes mellitus, and lack of exercise.[11] Interventions such as medications and lifestyle modifications to target these risk factors have improved mental clarity.[12]

Among lifestyle modifications, diet and nutrition play a major role in preventing Alzheimer's[13] and improving cognitive function. Specific nutritional interventions such as the Mediterranean-DASH Intervention for Neurodegenerative Delay (MIND) diet, which encourages leafy green vegetables, berries, beans, nuts, and fatty fish, such as salmon. The ketogenic diet also had positive effects.[14]

Several medications, such as aspirin and other anti-platelet drugs, are being prescribed by physicians to prevent secondary strokes in patients with vascular risk factors.[15] Yet these have not yet been proven to affect cognitive function.

That said, we know that patients diagnosed with a major occlusion, or blockage, in the carotid artery can benefit from surgery that
inserts a stent or small tube in the artery. Healthy carotid artery function is crucial because the carotid artery carries blood pumped from
the heart into the brain and other regions of the head. Surgery is often
recommended when carotid blood flows have fallen by 70 percent or
more, a condition known as *carotid artery stenosis.*

A study by Piegza et al., in 2021, showed that stenting of a blocked
carotid artery improved blood flows *and* cognitive function in patients
when assessments were made three months after the procedure.[16] None
of the patients in the first Piegza study had Alzheimer's symptoms, yet
later studies showed that the same stent surgery also improved cognitive functions in patients with cognitive decline.[17]

Ginkgo biloba extract (EGB761) is a medication often prescribed
for people with mild cognitive impairment and declining cognitive
skills related to narrowing blood flows in the brain. Known as Cere-
bonin, the drug has been shown to improve cognition, behavior, and
activities of daily living both in individuals with Alzheimer's and with
vascular dementia, but the biochemistry supporting these benefits
remains unknown.[18]

So far, medications designed to remove beta-amyloid plaques by
targeting them to cells (monoclonal antibodies) have failed to demonstrate significant cognitive improvement.[19]

Many medications have been developed to target Alzheimer's
other core biomarker, tau protein. The pharmaceutical designs of these
medications may involve one of the following: inhibition of kinases,
aggregation of tau, or stabilization of microtubules.

Tau protein has received increasing attention in recent years.[20]
Currently, most of the tau-targeting medications in clinical trials are
immunotherapies (active and passive immunizations). The hope is that
they will provide significant benefit.[21] Unfortunately, the first tau

immunization therapy studied on humans failed to show meaningful clinical improvement.[22]

Several supplements, such as curcumin, have been found to have anti-inflammatory and anti-amyloid effects.[23] However, these supplements have not been appropriately evaluated in prospective randomized clinical trials.

Dr. Michal Schwartz: Can the Brain's Immune System Defeat Alzheimer's?

Michal Schwartz is a pioneering researcher on the immune system's role in the health and repair of brain functions. Her immune therapies in mice studies have eliminated brain plaques associated with Alzheimer's disease and improved cognitive functions. Can they deliver similar results in humans? She may have the answers by the mid 2020s.

A professor of neuroimmunology at the Weizmann Institute of Science, Dr. Schwartz initiated several studies over the past quarter-century that collectively demonstrate how immune cells serve as guardians of brain health, essential for maintenance and repair throughout life.

She was the first to discover that macrophages (*Nature Medicine*, 1998) and T cells (*Nature Medicine*, 1999) carried in blood are needed to repair the central nervous system. She then established the immune system's unexpected yet fundamental role in supporting the brain's ability to grow and restructure its neural networks even as we age into our later years (*Nature Neuroscience*, 2006). Next, she suggested that dysfunctions in how brain cells and the immune system communicate are biochemical signs of an aging brain (*Science*, 2014).

Dr. Schwartz's research, undertaken mostly in the lab on animal models, defined how the brain together with immune cells discovered at its borders create an "ecosystem" that supports the brain's resilience. She theorized subsequently that the wearing down, or exhaustion, of the immune system plays a key role in perpetuating Alzheimer's disease, then asked this question: *Can we harness the immune system to treat Alzheimer's?*

The answer was yes—in mice. Her immune-based therapy eliminated brain plaques associated with the disease—and even restored the mice's cognitive abilities. In those studies, Dr. Schwartz found that an immune checkpoint blockade delivers three physiological benefits: (1) it targets the pathway of the programmed cell death protein 1 (PD-1); (2) it drives a systemic immune response that leads to activation of the CP for leukocyte trafficking; and (3) it reverses the sequence of biochemical breakdowns that cause Alzheimer's disease.

What is clear already is that Dr. Schwartz's novel approach marks a changing strategy for treating Alzheimer's. Broadly speaking, she is attempting, with immunotherapies, to treat the brain as a tissue, utilizing the same basic elements of physiology that apply to most tissues within our bodies.

Can HHP Prevent or Improve Alzheimer's?

We can say at this point that several factors in the advancing science around the molecular origins of Alzheimer's are known to reduce the odds that you, a loved one, or a friend will develop the disease.

What about the hyperoxic–hypoxic paradox? What we have established through current protocols and a history of healing or elevating cell activity in the brain is that HHP may indeed target some of the core elements responsible for the development and progression of Alzheimer's. But as we emphasized at the outset of this chapter, we have yet to prove this in randomized prospective clinical trials in humans.

Well then, what do we know that gives us hope that HHP may prove effective in curing or curtailing Alzheimer's? Consider these broad findings.

First, we know currently that HHP bolsters the normal health and functions of neurons by regenerating damaged neurons and stimulating growth of new neurons. HHP can induce angiogenesis. It can generate new blood vessels in the brain, a crucial element to restore and improve brain perfusion. HHP also repairs damage to the blood–brain barrier and reduces inflammation.

Next, HHP can improve the chemical efficiencies of cell life, reduce apoptosis, or abnormal volumes of cell death, and alleviate an imbalance between production and buildup of reactive oxygen species (ROS) and dampen the oxidative stress related to toxic aspects of ROS in cells and tissues.

Finally, we have also shown that HHP enhances the energy-converting functions of mitochondria in neurons and glial cells. HHP increases levels of neurotrophins, the proteins that help neurons survive and grow, and of nitric oxide, which helps blood vessels dilate, and improves brain and exercise performance.

While the efficacy of HBOT on the causes and effects of Alzheimer's disease has been studied mainly in animal models, we do have some anecdotal published reports from clinical cases on humans.

For example, a team of neurologists at Dalian Medical University in China concluded in 2020 that "based on previous studies and our recent findings . . . hyperbaric oxygen treatment may be a promising alternative therapy" for Alzheimer's, early-stage memory loss, and declines in other cognitive abilities (mild cognitive impairment).

The "recent findings" was a reference to their clinical study of eighty-three people, all with symptoms of progressing Alzheimer's. Forty-two had dementia, and eleven had early-stage memory problems, unable to recall normal activities such as appointments, conversations, or recent events. Another thirty had similar symptoms but did not receive HBOT treatments during the study.

The results showed significant improvement for participants with dementia and partial or total loss of memory in contrast to the control group. After one month of HBOT sessions, they had fewer problems with thinking and memory skills, attention and concentration, conceptual thinking, and other cognitive skills. Participants with Alzheimer's also scored higher in their ability to manage their own daily living activities on assessments made one and three months after the HBOT sessions were completed.

Our Ambitious Study of Early-Stage Alzheimer's

We hope to determine in the next few years how effective HHP might be in halting and reversing these breakdowns in metabolism. We at the Sagol Center are running what will now be one of the most comprehensive clinical studies for prodromal Alzheimer's—patients with mild cognitive impairment who have evidence of amyloid protein deposits in their brains.

The research will include months of follow-up, brain imaging, computerized cognitive testing, blood biomarkers, and interviews to assess changes triggered by the therapy. One of Israel's largest health insurance companies, Maccabi Healthcare Services, is collaborating with us on this study. We estimate it will take as many as three years to complete. The first steps were underway in early 2023.

In summary, ischemia is a common trigger for several neurodegenerative diseases, including Alzheimer's disease. The narrowing or interruption of blood flows contributes to chronic ischemia in brain tissue, accumulation of beta-amyloid and tau proteins, inflammation of neurons with glial activation, loss of neurons, damage to the blood–brain barrier, and dysfunction of mitochondria.

For all these reasons, and keeping in mind the huge, accelerating financial burden Alzheimer's is imposing on societies now, we must make slowing and reversing ischemia a major priority in neurology and medical science. We already have many advanced weapons to prevent this armageddon. We just need to employ and continue to develop them.

As I see it, our major task as physicians and scientists in industrialized Western nations is to do our best to generate the science and medical interventions that one day will enable us to achieve a healthier, Alzheimer's-free society.

Key Takeaways

1. Ischemia, or reduced blood flow, is a common trigger for several neurodegenerative diseases, including Alzheimer's disease.
2. We might be able to slow or reverse the natural progression of dementia and Alzheimer's if we can intervene sooner to prevent narrowing blood flows in the brain.
3. The presence of beta-amyloid proteins in the brain is *not sufficient on its own* to predict with certainty that a patient eventually will develop Alzheimer's disease. Beta-amyloid is not the primary cause of the common type of Alzheimer's. Many clinical drug trials targeting beta-amyloid and tau proteins in various forms have failed to induce meaningful improvement in cognitive skills.
4. Targeting the tissue with immune therapies and inducing regeneration by HBOT in mice studies has eliminated brain plaques associated with Alzheimer's disease and improved cognitive functions. Can they deliver similar results in humans? Time will tell . . .

PART III

THE EVOLUTION OF AGING

CHAPTER 11

Aging Is a Good Thing

If you could choose which age you would rather be, would you want to be eighteen or seventy years old?

Are you laughing at the thought? In my experience, most people do.

To them, the answer seems so obvious: "I would want to be eighteen, of course. You are healthier, stronger physically, more sexually attractive, and probably more socially active. Your mind is more alert, more curious. You are just coming into your own, making decisions about the life you want and how to build that life. It's an exciting time, blooming with challenges and promise."

"By the time you are seventy, if you've lived that long, your health is declining or in doubt; you may have cancer, heart disease, Alzheimer's disease, or other chronic ailments. Your eyesight, hearing, and memory are fading. If you are working, it's probably because you need the money. Some of your friends and family members are dead. Most of all, you yourself don't have much longer to live! Who would want to be seventy?"

Creators of the immensely popular TV sitcom *Friends* tapped into a similar celebratory zeitgeist around the coming of age. The show would be "about sex, love, relationships, careers, a time in your life when everything's possible."[1]

But what if we could put aside that anticipated deterioration of our body, of the wondrous yet ultimately fragile biology that each of us inhabits as humans? What then? Aging would be embraced as a good thing, not a bleak thing.

Many good things happen as we age. You gain more knowledge and life experience. You have relationships with your family, your children are already grown and likely have become independent, you have more colleagues and old friends. You may well have more economic resources at seventy than eighteen, with a higher income and more savings.

Who would choose to be eighteen years old with limited financial resources and limited knowledge and wisdom accumulated from your education, work, and life experience—*if* . . . and this is now becoming possible . . . *if* you could have the same potent biological functions you had at age eighteen when you are seventy? *And* that with this enduring, steady health, your prospects for many more years of active, healthy experiences still lie ahead?

Aging and *old* are not the same thing. You are old if your general health and your mental and physical vibrancy are weak and failing. You are old if you continuously look back and relive the past and are not really making plans for the future. You are old if you are not actively engaged in making yourself useful to others.

Aging and old are not the same thing.

The difference lies in performance—both mental and physical performance. This choice is not a fantasy. You can retain or rebuild the vibrant health of your heart, brain, kidneys, liver, and other bodily organs as well as the rest of your body you enjoyed during your early years. And, at the same time, you and others can benefit from the wisdom, knowledge, and life skills you have gathered as you age into your seventies.

Biological Bottlenecks

The main question from the perspective of medical science is whether your biology is declining or not. This depends to a large degree on the balance between those things that impair the smooth workings of our youthful biology—we call these the *degenerative factors*—and those things that renew and restore our youthful biology—our regenerative and repair capabilities. As we go through life, our systems naturally encounter types of bottlenecks, misfirings, or erosions that cause our body's repair mechanisms to fade from their high points of performance to low ones.

The goal for us as humans and the goal for our medical, nutritional, and fitness advisers should be to unclog these bottlenecks and reset the balance toward positive regeneration—all those things that renew and restore our youthful biology. The technology is still developing, but we have reached a point where we can already mark them. We can identify where and how these bottlenecks have emerged among our trillions of cells, and then apply our advancing, intricate knowledge of microbiology to remove them.

The challenge for physicians and medical scientists then becomes a never-ending one. But that's the beauty of it all. When we successfully remove one bottleneck, we create opportunities for new ones to emerge. For example, one reason that Alzheimer's disease today afflicts greater numbers of people later in life is because more people live longer; the average age in the United States has risen in the past one hundred years to 76.6 years in 2021 from 60.9 years in 1921.[2]

When we are young, we have an amazing physiology, an amazing ability to regenerate trillions of cells as our bodies grow through our teens and, for some, into our twenties. Most of us continue to enjoy this physical vibrancy throughout our twenties. Once into our forties, our capacity to regenerate cells and tissue begins to decline.

Consider the life cycle of our blood vessels. Over time, the inner walls accumulate materials, such as plaque, that narrow our blood vessels and impair blood flows. (Plaque consists of deposits of fatty substances, cholesterol, cellular waste, calcium, and fibrin.) This is *atherosclerosis*, a hardening of the arteries.

Occlusion in aging blood vessels reduces supplies of oxygen and energy to cells and tissue wherever these blood vessels reach. Statins are prescribed for millions of people to slow plaque buildup in veins and arteries. Anti-coagulants, such as aspirin and other drugs, are prescribed to reduce the odds of the plaque rupturing and producing a blood clot in blood vessels or the heart.

When one of those blood vessels' destination is the brain, and an occlusion happens abruptly, such as when plaque is torn, a sudden loss of consciousness happens. If the occlusion expands slowly over time, this condition gradually impairs our mental sharpness and we experience cognitive decline. When an occlusion in blood vessels nourishing the heart accumulates slowly over time, we call it *cardiac functional decline*. If not checked, this eventually may cause heart failure.

Aging Starts in the Embryo

The conventional modern view during the past generation has been that aging starts somewhere in our fifties or sixties, and on average we will live into our mid or late seventies.

Our perspective as physicians of enhanced medicine is different. We see aging as an ongoing process that starts from the day we are created at conception when the female egg is fertilized by the male sperm. Aging begins after our mothers have delivered us from a fetus swelling in their uterus out into this world. We can separate the aging process into three major, well-defined biological periods:

1. Development and growth
2. Reproductive
3. Post-reproductive

When we are young, during development and growth, our regenerative capacity is high. We have a wonderful physical capability, healthy blood vessels, and an abundance of potent stem cells that can easily replicate and differentiate as needed to transform themselves into any of the trillions of specific cells that are damaged or missing in our bodies as we age. The net effect is that we build and repair tissue rapidly. If our skin is cut or a bone is broken, the repair in our early years happens rapidly. The age span for this first period runs typically from birth into our mid or late teens.

The reproductive period for a woman begins by her mid teens and continues well into her forties. For a man, it's from the mid teens into his eighties. During our reproductive period, our biology continues to have a relatively good balance between the regenerative and the degenerative capacities, so the net effect is a balanced biology. Nature wants to preserve us during this time because we are producing the next generation for this world.

The post-reproductive period is where our biology really needs help. During this period, unfortunately, the imbalance is striking. Regenerative capabilities decline drastically. The degeneration of our biology continues. The net effect is decline, depletion, and regression.

Why is that?

The most common denominators of biological bottlenecks related to aging are: stem cells, "pipes" (the respiratory airways), circulatory (blood vessels carrying blood to and from the heart), and the gastrointestinal track that collectively deliver oxygen and nourishment to our body and remove waste.

Stem Cells

Let's pause here for a moment to appreciate again the astounding qualities of stem cells and how the body creates, deploys, and heals itself with stem cells.

As I just intimated, our entire body is created from two cells, sperm from the male and ovule from the female. This pairing creates an omnipotent stem cell, one from which every other cell as well as every piece of tissue and every organ in our body is generated. Stem cells do two remarkable things: they can precisely replicate their biological structures, and they can "print" bespoke three-dimensional repair kits to heal damaged tissue. Our evolutionary path recognized—or, if you prefer, whoever created us knew—that our planetary environments teem with bacteria, viruses, and other threats to our human biology and our survival. There were going to be problems.

Nature did give us the ability to regenerate an entire liver, but not every organism in our bodies. There are a few species that can do this. Salamanders, planarians, and the Mexican axolotl are examples. In the big picture, though, we humans go through life without spare parts. Yet animals might one day provide humans a plethora of spare parts. The recipient of the first pig-to-human heart transplant survived two months in 2022 before the pig heart was rejected. A second patient at the University of Maryland Medical Center lived five weeks after similar surgery in 2023 for a pig-heart transplant. Today humans provide each other with spare parts in limited ways such as bone marrow, kidneys, livers, and heart transplants.

Stem cells fill that gap, at least partially. Nature has given our bodies a three-dimensional printer that churns out perfect models of cells we need to continuously replace dead and dying cells. You probably don't give much if any thought to your microbiological renewal, but you should know that every three months or so, aging cells existing throughout our bodies are replaced. Your molecular biology is constantly being regenerated. In that sense, you are an entirely different physical being! You don't see or sense this when all is well because DNA sequences of new cells exactly match those of discarded cells.

Stem cells are dormant until a specific trigger causes them to vigorously copy themselves (replication), move through the bloodstream (migrate), or precisely duplicate the structure and function of cells in specific tissues where repairs are needed (differentiation). Moreover, new blood vessels are created when energy and stem cells are combined with the specific trigger (angiogenesis). New blood vessels are essential. They carry nutrition, stem cells, immune cells, and blood cells with increased capacity to carry oxygen. All of these create harmonious chords in the body's regenerative process. All are needed to improve tissue functionality or to protect specific tissue from further damage.

During our developmental and growth period, our bodies possess a huge number of stem cells. Regeneration is dominant. The net effect of this bounty is biological and physical growth as our bodies mature into adulthood.

By the end of our reproductive years, we reach a kind of steady state, a balance between our regenerative capabilities and our degenerative processes. The degenerative elements actually take command during our post-reproductive period.

Looking across all three periods, you can see how our ability to regenerate cells and tissue declines. Put another way, the biology of our systems gradually weakens until an acceleration of degenerative processes largely overtakes regenerative capabilities late in our post-reproductive period.

This is nature's way. Living species are designed by evolution to breed the next generation, and to die when they can procreate no longer. If you are not bringing a new generation into the world, you are disposable to nature. Except for humans, *homo sapiens*. We are the only species on Earth that continues to live long after our reproductive years have waned. We did not become the rulers of this world by chance.

The reason, which we will explore in more detail shortly, is that for us, there is immense value in the knowledge and wisdom that our elders accumulate through their lifetimes. This valuable, acquired wisdom is what constantly improves the knowledge, prosperity, and resilience of children, the younger generation. As members of each new generation emerge, they apply elders' knowledge to their own lives and then, adding to that knowledge, pass it on to their children. Elders not only bring the new generation into the world. They educate them to make their lives and their world a better place.

"Pipes"

When we are children, our pipes—our circulatory systems—are fresh; they're pristine, clear, and flexible. As we grow into adulthood, as we just noted, the effects of slowly building corrosion begin to appear in our blood vessels. Plaque builds up along interior artery walls. If there is too much plaque, arterial walls stiffen and reduce blood flow pumped by the heart. Our pipes become corroded. This process, atherosclerosis, deprives cells and tissues throughout the body of oxygen and nutrients. Chronic age-related diseases, such as heart disease, cognitive decline, ineffective erection in men, and many other age-related diseases are the result of this dreaded atherosclerosis.

Aging also happens within our cells. For example, during their lifetime, cells will replicate about forty times and then stop. Nothing more. This in effect is the cell's genomic clock. Once cells stop replicating, their function is suboptimal, not as designed. But our biology responds magnificently to these setbacks. Once a cell is no longer functioning optimally, it is expected to go through an organized cell death process (the medical term is *apoptosis)* that sets the stage for nonfunctioning cells to be cleaned from the system. This cleansing process helps prevent damage to surrounding healthy cells, to the organs' systems, and to our whole organism.

Senescent Cells and Telomeres

Sometimes failing cells don't kill themselves through apoptosis. They become "zombie" cells—simply limp, not functioning cells. But they are not dead. They just remain in situ, growing old. All the while, the risk of changes in their molecular structure can harm healthy cells nearby. Known as *senescent cells,* they become stuck—and can become a real problem if they accumulate in our bodies; this is what happens to most people.

Senescent cells can induce inflammation. Worse yet, they can accumulate mutations and become cancer cells. Senescent cells are like garbage that remains inside your house that becomes smelly and toxic if not removed. We often find the footprints, or markers, of senescent cells in many chronic age-related diseases.

"Cellular senescence is a response of an individual cell to stress," explains Laura Niedernhofer, a biochemist and physician whose research has demonstrated how senescent cells accumulate damaged

---

* *Senescent* is an adjective defined by *Merriam-Webster* as something associated with being old or in the process of aging.

DNA and cause disease.[3] These cells send signals to attract immune cells to clear them away, but as more senescent cells accumulate, the immune system, also aging, can become overwhelmed. "This leads to a state of chronic inflammation that we believe is one of the hallmarks of aging" and can make you vulnerable to several diseases common in old age.

A cell's DNA is protected each time the DNA strand divides by bumpers at the ends of the cell's double strands. The bumpers, called *telomeres*, are like the caps or tips at the end of shoelaces that bind and protect the lace ends from fraying. These telomeres help keep the DNA intact as new cells are replicated precisely (in most cases) from the originals. Telomeres are essential players in the body's spectacular ballet of molecular regeneration.

But with each cell division, telomeres lose small bits of their coding and become shorter. They become like a precision machine tool that loses its sharp edge over time. When telomeres that help replicate the cells' DNA become too short, cells can go into what Elissa Epel, co-author of an authoritative book on telomeres, calls "cell-cycle arrest."[4] Most often, instead of dying, shortened telomeres themselves become old senescent cells.

"When the telomeres start screaming out signals—'We're too short! Watch out! We could become a cancer cell!'—it becomes a nonfunctioning senescent cell that secretes inflammation," Epel says.[5]

Neuroscientist Daniel J. Levitin has a simple way of explaining this. "When scientists talk about aging, we're not talking about chronological age, because there is a wide variety of ways that people age. What we're really interested in is the accumulated effect of things that happen to our bodies that cause difficulties. Neuroscientists use the word *senescence*—just a fancy Latin-rooted word that means to grow old or to age. You can't do anything to turn back your chronological age, but you can decrease the likelihood of senescence by adopting simple practices."[6]

If we could perfect a way to slow the shortening of telomeres or even transform shortening telomeres to an optimal length, that insight could be a breakthrough for lowering the prevalence of chronic disease associated with aging. More people would be healthier living into or beyond their eighties, and they would be able to contribute more to their families, neighbors, and communities. We are closing in on this breakthrough.

Our clinic in Israel has demonstrated how to lengthen telomeres in humans and at the same time reduce the presence of senescent cells in our bodies. (You'll recall from chapter 2 that the length of Avishai Abrahami's telomeres increased by nearly 47 percent.) We were the first in the world to do this.

Turning Back the Biological Clock

What can we do now to turn back the biological clock? Based on the scientific knowledge we have today, as we saw in chapter 1, four crucial elements are needed:

1. Nurturing forward-looking aspirations (knowing your purpose in life)
2. Inducing beneficial levels of positive stress in our physiology, such as through intermittent fasting, exercise, challenging our mental capacities, or undertaking intellectual projects (hormesis)
3. Taking daily supplements of prescribed metformin that target mitochondrial functioning
4. Inducing the biochemical spark for abundant production of stem cells, mitochondria, and generation of new blood vessels (hypoxia-induced factor)

The best prevention for age-related functional decline is to make yourself needed by others. Making yourself "need-able" is the catchword I use with patients. *Are you need-able? Do you wake up in the morning with some purpose, some commitment to use your skills and experience to connect and help others?* You must have a plan for the future, and it must be *your* plan for the future.

Hormesis

Again, as we saw in chapter 1, hormesis is a grand idea and a grand bargain. The idea is to expose your body to a specific stress in low "doses"—in a safe, controlled way that does not approach some higher level that could cause real damage. The bargain is to push yourself, to induce stress in limited amounts that will tune your body, not damage it, and prepare it for specific physical challenges you might encounter.

Let's take intermittent fasting as an example. When we abstain from eating, typically for ten to thirteen hours, our cells devour the best source of nutrients available to it—that is, until food is consumed again. That best available source is senescent cells or dead cells still in our system. The more we eliminate these "garbage" cells from our system, the more we reduce the risk of cancers and other diseases. Fasting helps us "eat" the garbage that otherwise accumulates at the molecular level. In medical terms, this process is called *autophagy*. Autophagy is one of the most important, and rarely exploited, levers we have to slow biological aging. You get the idea from the ancient Greek words from which autophagy is derived: *autophagos*, or "self-devouring," and *kytos*, meaning "hollow."

Intermittent fasting also helps reduce fat. After eight to twelve hours of no calories, your blood is low on sugar, your liver is empty of sugar, and your muscle cells are empty of sugar because you feed your brain through the night as you sleep. The average brain weighs 3 pounds (2 percent of our average body weight), but it consumes 20 percent of our energy. Where will your brain get the energy it needs to carry on while you sleep? The answer is that the brain mobilizes the fat surrounding your stomach and other abdominal organs because this is where those last calories reside—in the visceral fat. Over time, as you fast intermittently, you lose that fat.

The drills and disciplines of physical fitness are other examples of how our bodies benefit from hormesis. Let's briefly recall here two points mentioned in chapter 1: First, physical exercise builds more mitochondria, more muscles, and more blood vessels. It improves your heart's capacity to pump more blood through the body, enabling your mitochondria to process more oxygen and to generate more energy. Second, when you exercise, direct benefits flow immediately from your body's natural biochemistry throughout your body. For example, exercise may directly affect areas of the brain such as the amygdala and prefrontal cortex that are rich in receptors for endocannabinoids. Endocannabinoids regulate stress and immune responses as well as critical functions such as learning, memory, and sleep and enable us to sort out our emotions.

Metformin

After it was first approved for use in the United States in 1995, metformin was prescribed mostly for Type 2 diabetes because it lowered glucose levels. It now may be the best available drug for turning back the biological clock.

In recent years, a flurry of new studies has shown significant benefits from metformin in reducing the chronic diseases of aging. When patients with severe sepsis infection were treated with metformin in our own intensive care unit in Israel, they had a much better chance of recovery than those who did not have metformin. Metformin reduces the risks of cancers and heart disease. It helps produce more energy in diabetes patients and lowers glucose. It is the only drug known to help diabetes patients live longer.

Scientists have not yet fully described the precise biochemical mechanism (or mechanisms) for how metformin achieves these outcomes. Its genes have the rare characteristic of determining more than one trait of an organism. That feature, referred to as *pleiotropic*, may hold the answer. Today we do understand that metformin exerts many of its actions through the ways mitochondria are regenerated.

Metformin also helps mitochondria function with less "waste," such as the reactive oxygen species that can create cell damage. It helps reduce cell deaths caused by mitochondrial malfunctions, such as those related to Type 2 diabetes. Metformin may also inhibit cancer cell growth and proliferation, according to recent studies, at least partly through its beneficial effects on mitochondria. Moreover, it triggers autophagy, cleaning out senescent and dead cells.

Many medical scientists who study the biology of aging, people I know and respect, take metformin regularly. I've considered it as well but have decided not to take it at this stage. I don't want to modify my mitochondria by ingesting a chemical from the outside. I prefer to bolster the performance of my mitochondria and all the benefits they provide through fasting, exercise, and HHP. That said, I certainly will keep metformin on my short list of intriguing pharmaceutical options for a later time in my life, perhaps several decades from now.

Longevity Lessons of Bowhead Whales

Nature has given humans a majestic model within the family of marine mammals for extraordinary health and longevity—the bowhead whale.

Bowhead whales are believed to be the longest-living mammal, with lifespans known to be 200 years or more. A genome sequence analysis by Australia's national science agency has put the maximum lifespan of bowhead whales at 268 years! The more important point for us here is that bowhead whales are remarkably healthy creatures. They have an unusually high resistance to cancer and other aging diseases despite their long lives and prodigious physical dimensions—an average length of eighty feet and average weight above eighty tons.

Their observable patterns of daily activity check the boxes of at least three of those four elements we noted for turning back the biological clock.

1. **Hyperoxic–hypoxic paradox/hypoxia-inducible factor and exercise.** Bowhead whales typically dive for approximately twenty minutes (and sometimes up to an hour) from the surface of frigid waters in their Arctic habitat to feed on schools of fish, then they rise to the surface to breathe air. The repeated fluctuation in oxygen and pressure generates HIF.

2. **A diet mainly of fish and intermittent fasting.** Food restriction and fasting during the winter typically last three months, which promotes autophagy on a grand scale. During fasting, the whales are inactive and rarely eat. Instead, they are cleaning out the garbage when their metabolism turns to consuming dead and senescent cells for nourishment after the daily intake of fresh fish is long past.

3. **Hormesis.** Patterns of constant motion and frequent deep diving are fitness drills in effect that activate all muscles, trigger mitochondria, and burn massive

amounts of energy. Bowhead whales are not fast swim-
mers. When threatened by smaller, more propulsive
killer whales, a principal aquatic predator, they seek
shallow waters for safety. Humans have been lethal
predators as well, and we are the number one threat to
their longevity. Bowhead whales were hunted aggres-
sively into the early twentieth century before governments imposed whaling restrictions.

Do bowhead whales also check a fourth box: Have a purpose?
Quite possibly. Bowheads are known for intense, playful sprees of
social group interactions—tail and flipper slapping and out-of-water
breaching. Like many baleen whales, they communicate underwater
through sound. Normally found in groups of three, they can congre-
gate in larger numbers where food is abundant and during migration
jaunts. Females' birthing years begin when they are roughly twenty-five
years old and typically follow cycles of only one calf every three to
seven years. Mating is assumed to occur around March. Gestation
typically is thirteen or fourteen months.

Bowhead whales' social communications give us clues that they
also live with a purpose, but we can only speculate. Where do we draw
a line between instinct and will? The instinct theory of motivation
holds that instinct drives all behaviors in all forms of life. We have yet
to create neurological and observational tools we would need to truly
get inside the heads of bowhead whales.

Unhealthy Diets, Lower Life Expectancy

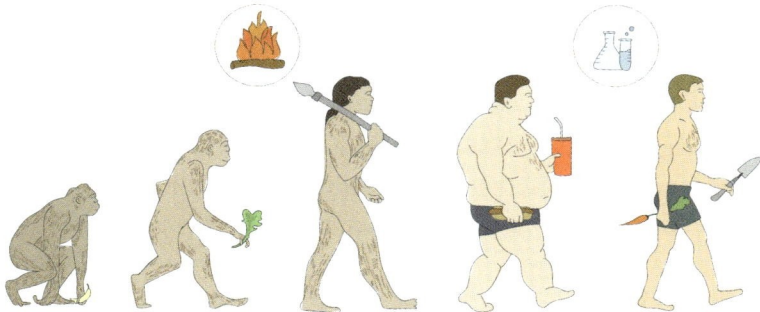

What signature advance thousands of years ago enabled *homo sapiens* to dominate other animals and rule the planet? When we learned to control fire. Controlling fire opened the gate to cooking meat and other food, which reduced the amount of energy required to digest food. Think about how you feel after eating a large meal with meat. You feel like sleeping. That's because more energy is diverted to the intestinal tract for digestion, and less to the brain.

Our evolving biology exploited the excess energy created within us by growing and developing larger brains, specifically the outer layer of gray matter, the cortex, where many of our higher cognitive functions reside. Neurons there equip us at the cellular level for decision-making, motivation, attention, learning, memory, problem-solving, and conceptual thinking, as well as our increasing capacity to imagine the future, plan, and move about. As the dimensions of the human brain expanded, so did the capacities that enabled us to become superior communicators and problem solvers.

But in the last hundred years or so, our deteriorating eating habits, dominated by so-called fast foods, began taking control over the diet that brought us to where we are today. The rise in obesity, diabetes, cardiovascular disease, cognitive decline, and cancers has been obvious for decades.

The costs of treating these diseases are already a burden on government budgets. Instead of adopting the best and simplest form of treatment—changing our diets, we are pushed to take commercial drugs designed to reduce some of the side effects created by the toxic materials we eat. Projections for higher percentages of people suffering from obesity and diabetes seem certain to drive treatment costs higher for those diseases alone.

These diet-driven health breakdowns have contributed to the alarming decline in average lifespan in the United States since 2019. The damage of high-carb diets to our organs and circulatory systems is well documented, but we should not overlook or discount how poor eating habits damage our brains. Eating bad food damages our physiology and our mental capacities.

We have trillions of organisms in our bodies tied to thousands of species, a collection of organisms called *microbiota*. The bacterium within our microbiota is a mix of beneficial and harmful organisms. If the ratio of harmful bacteria rises beyond our systems' ability to contain their negative effects, that harmful bacteria deliver signals to the brain that can degrade the healthy functions of all our organs, including the brain.

In their informative, solidly researched book *The Good Gut: Taking Control of Your Weight, Your Mood, and Your Long-Term Health,* Stanford University microbiology and immunology researchers Erica Sonnenburg and Justin Sonnenburg broke new ground in 2015 in our understanding of brain–gut connections.[7]

They describe an "information superhighway" comprised of a network of hundreds of millions of neurons and a highway of chemicals and hormones "that constantly provide feedback about how hungry we are, whether or not we're experiencing stress, or if we've ingested a disease-causing microbe." In this way, microbiota also help the immune system differentiate between good and bad microbes, including disease-causing microbes.

"Recent evidence indicates that not only is our brain 'aware' of our gut microbes, but these bacteria can influence our perception of the world and alter our behavior. It is becoming clear that the influence of our microbiota reaches far beyond the gut to affect an aspect of our biology few would have predicted—our mind."

Key Takeaways

1. We should think of aging as a lifelong biological process that starts the day we are born, one that we can influence significantly to live healthier for longer.
2. We often find markers of senescent cells, which can induce inflammation, in chronic age-related diseases. HBOT enables many of these cells to recover much of their healthy functions.
3. Telomeres help keep DNA intact as new cells replicate precisely (in most cases) from the originals, but telomeres shorten, or wear out, over time. Our clinic in Israel has demonstrated how to lengthen telomeres and at the same time reduce the presence of senescent cells in our bodies.

CHAPTER 12

Retirement Is a Bad Thing

Medical scientists have conducted countless studies demonstrating how biological decline accelerates when people retire from their working life. I see this all the time in my medical practice, and later in this chapter, I'll give you a few examples.

Friedrich Nietzsche, the nineteenth-century German philosopher who embraced self-reliance, reasoned that if you have a "why," you can withstand any "how."[1] Nietzsche had it right. I push people whose sense of purpose is foggy or absent, whose physical abilities are failing, to define their "why."

Make Yourself Need-Able

I suppose I am not your typical physician. When someone asks me to take them on as a patient, I don't look first at their medical history. I always ask them, "What do you do? How do you spend your days?" If the response suggests they are adrift, with no purpose or mission that pulls them forward regardless of whatever they accomplished before, I stop.

"Go make a plan and bring it back to me," I tell them. "Otherwise, I will not treat you."

Some may think this attitude violates my Hippocratic oath, my responsibilities to heal. I don't. With many patients, this command to find a purpose in your life is the best cure I can offer. Allow me to explain.

The best cure for age-related functional decline is to make yourself needed by others. To have a purpose. Find something that you need to wake up for in the morning. Something that will give you purpose, meaning. I've learned that whatever cures I might effect in someone's body will be temporary if they have no plans for the future.

One day years ago, a talented engineer who developed advanced rockets came to meet with me about a year after he left his work. He was in his early sixties. After his retirement, he had been walking on the beach every morning, swimming with friends. Relaxing.

Being an elite engineer, he sensed though that his mental clarity and physical resilience were weakening. Small viruses now made him sick. Several doctors he had consulted could not help him. From our first conversation, I could tell he was lost, drifting. He no longer had an all-consuming challenge to match the remarkable missions that had defined his career.

So, I offered one. By chance, a startup company I am involved with was stymied at the time in developing new technologies for intubating patients in intensive care wards. "I have the best cure for you," I told him. "What?!?" he replied. "We need an engineer with significant experience to help us on an important project. If we succeed, medical professionals will be able to give better care to critically ill patients. We'll save lives. You'll help save lives."

He accepted my offer, my treatment. Since then—for more than a decade—he has been fully absorbed in helping the company overcome a succession of engineering challenges to improve the quality and functioning of ventilators. Countless patients in ICUs have benefited, recovering their health and living longer.

"Where Are You? We Need You."

The day after my former professor and department head was forced to retire at age sixty-five, his life changed dramatically. He had been responsible for seriously ill patients in addition to educating residents and medical students, taking calls all day, making difficult decisions that could save lives . . . or not.

Suddenly those demands went away. He thought the computer must not be working; he was not receiving emails. The cellular phone must be broken; no one was calling him. Then he heard my voice coming through the handset. "I need you," I said to him. "I need your help. I want you to help me advise and train the residents." He was so thankful. After taking a week off, he came to see me for his assignments. "Shai, I am so happy you called me," he said.

None of the professors I know ever want to retire. Their work gives them meaning.

My father came to Israel from Morocco. He had to drop out of high school when he was fifteen to work full time to help his father—my grandfather, a farmer—support the family. So, my father became a landscape gardener, working with lumber and other materials as well as plantings to construct what often were quite elaborate designs.

From the time I was a young boy, I worked, first in the fields with my grandfather, and then after I was thirteen alongside my father until I went into the military when I was eighteen.

My father's gardening life was strenuous; it was more like construction labor. Digging. Lifting. Building. Hard labor under a hot sun. When he reached sixty-seven, he retired. *Why not?* he reasoned. After all those years, he now could stop because he would have enough income from Israel's social pension.

On the day after my father retired, I pleaded with him, "You know, daddy. I love you so much. You have to work. If needed, I will pay your salary. But you need to work. Otherwise, I will become totally busy *treating you!*"

I was serious, but he laughed this off. Around that time, though, he had a stroke, then cardiac surgery. He recovered, fortunately, and for more than a decade now he has taken my advice. He works, not with the same intensity as before, but he is need-able.

Now in his early eighties, he starts the day at six o'clock walking outside, exercising in the gym, playing Ping-Pong, and eating breakfast with the guys, then he works six to eight hours as a supervisor for a landscaping company with big private and government projects. It's work he enjoys, peacefully. He feels needed. If he skips a day, he will get calls. "Where are you? We need you," they say. He has never been hospitalized for any ailment since that first year after he retired.

Unless you are needed in the world, the universe does not invest in you; specifically, the durability of your biology. In the wild, when animals age chronologically, they die or are eaten by predators. For humans it is different.

"Never Grow Old. Never Ever Die Young."

As we age, our knowledge and insights about the past and present are valued by younger generations. They rely on elders to help them prepare for the future. Yet, if you believe you are not needed by anyone, if you believe you have no value for generations today and tomorrow, then you are wasting the resources of nature. Your biology will break down. Cancer, heart disease, Alzheimer's disease, and so on.

There is no question we are going to die. Dying is not a choice, not for any forms of life on Earth. We all will die. But being old? We can die without being old. That's the goal.

James Taylor had the mantra about right when the iconic American singer–songwriter and musician first sang this about the human spirit: "Never give up, never slow down, never grow old, never ever die young."

In my view, a person is old when they only look to the past to "what I used to do." Young people look to the future and ask, "What am I going to do?"

Chronological age is irrelevant. I have had patients come to me "old" at age thirty-five. Others were "young" at age ninety-two. If you have plans, if you are looking to the future to make an impact, you are young. If you have no plans, you are old.

Once on the same day, two highly talented retired men came to me for consultations. One was an amazing engineer and pilot who had suffered a heart attack after he stopped working in his late fifties. His staggering mental abilities and physical strength were fading.

After him a successful entrepreneur came in and sat in the same chair. In his mid-fifties, he had built several companies and made millions through public stock offerings. He didn't need to work to earn a living, so he didn't. His brain, physical, and sexual functions were all in decline. To both, I said, "My friend, I will treat you. But first, you have to find something to work for. A mission. Come back to me with a plan."

Raise the Retirement Age

We all should have the privilege to continue working, to stay active. Most of us start working when we are young because we need to earn a living. Later in life, we need to keep working because it is essential for our well-being, our connection to others. When this privilege is ignored or taken away, the beginning of a medical tragedy can quickly take shape. This tragedy is one we can and should be able to avoid and be obligated to help others avoid.

The best medical intervention to stop this epidemic of post-retirement diseases has nothing to do with hospitals, clinics, pharmaceuticals, or consultations with physicians or nurses. It should be public policy: we should raise the qualifying age for public pensions. Raise the retirement age. Change the definition of "old." I'll say it again: **There is no question we're going to die. Dying is not a choice. But being old? This is a choice we can make for ourselves.**

If I chaired the U.S. Food & Drug Administration, I would immediately urge the U.S. Congress to raise the retirement age to seventy-five from sixty-seven. Then, after a few years, when the advancing science of enhanced medicine can further support the overall health of the nation's aging population, raise it again into the eighties. The best treatment for reducing or delaying multiple chronic diseases related to aging is to raise the retirement age. Once governments define a retirement age, societies become stuck.

The accepted modern view about aging and retirement has its origins in policies introduced in the nineteenth century. In 1887, German Chancellor Otto von Bismarck set *seventy* as the qualifying age for a government-funded pension. Back then the average life expectancy for Germans from birth was just under *forty* years.

Germany was the first country to create a public pension system. The German parliament lowered the age to sixty-five in 1913. Two decades later—six years into the Great Depression, the U.S. Congress followed Germany, setting the retirement age at sixty-five as part of the Social Security Act in 1935. Five years into the Depression, average

U.S. life expectancy was sixty-two; more than 50 percent of American men sixty-five or older lived in poverty.

The first months after retirement is a time someone's biology often begins to crash. I see this time after time in my medical practice, in patient after patient. Maybe you know people like this and can encourage them toward a new sense of mission and purpose.

Some retired men come to me after other physicians are not able to help them with the decline in mental and physical abilities they experienced, including impotence. Decline in sexual function often is a serious incentive to seek medical advice.* Yet some men will initially protest after I urge them to return to work. "I have enough money; I don't need to work. I don't want to work. My job was so stressful; I needed to retire."

Fighter Pilot, Professor

One of these patients was a much-decorated Israeli fighter pilot. Back in civilian life, for decades he worked long days and nights, building a highly profitable company. He made a fortune, then retired abruptly at age fifty. It wasn't long before he suffered a heart attack. For the next six years, as he explained to me, his mental and physical prowess was in a steady gradual decline. His capacity for sexual relations became negligible. Sitting across from me, I could sense his fear of biological aging, of death. Despite all his amazing gifts and talents, he was despondent.

---

* In my speeches at conferences and coaching sessions with physicians, I often encourage them to ask patients if they have any concerns or questions about their sexual performance. Most physicians stay away from initiating a discussion about sex, but I have found repeatedly that patients are eager to talk about it. Many thank me for opening the door to that conversation, saying they had never had a physician do this for them before.

"You don't need to work at the same stress level you were used to in the past," I assured him, "but you must have some passion, some motivation, that pulls you outward as you awake fully in the morning. Start a second career. Become a volunteer. Start or join a project for a community, for certain people, for whatever you want. It doesn't matter. Write your plan down and bring it to me. *You don't need the money; you need the gratitude.* You must be 'need-able.' Who needs you? I need to see what you are going to do. Otherwise, I will not treat you."

Raising the retirement age is a pressing economic issue as well as a medical imperative. So is reducing healthcare's bulging share of national economies.

As more people live longer, no government will be able to afford paying public pensions and medical costs at current levels.[†]

As Social Security and other entitlement programs drain the Treasury of tax revenues, less money will be available to fund urgent needs such as rebuilding bridges and highways, supporting preschool and school lunch programs and medical research, or combating cyber threats.

Key Takeaways

1. Old is a state of mind for people who are living in the past with no productive plans or goals ahead of them.
2. Make yourself "need-able" in your community or society; need-able for other people or in pursuit of a specific goal. Once you have this mindset, we can help with your biology.

---

† The U.S. federal debt amounted to more than $33 trillion in 2023. That equaled a staggering 130 percent of total U.S. economic output in 2022.

3. The gap between how well and how long elite performers live is going to accelerate, in contrast to people with poor diets and fitness habits who are creating conditions for chronic age-related diseases.

4. We can expect the magnitude of elite performers' contributions to society and future generations to keep expanding.

CHAPTER 13

My Personal Regimen: HBOT, Fitness, Nutrition, and Diet

That first HBOT study we conducted with stroke patients that I recounted in chapter 5 was so convincing, I thought, *My God, these results are amazing. I need the HBOT for me.*

Since then, for sixteen years, I have repeated the full HBOT protocol with sixty sessions every two years and sometimes sooner. I want to keep challenging my mental sharpness, so for maintenance I spend two hours in the chamber once or twice a week.

My cognitive and physiological data today at age fifty-three are much better than sixteen years ago. Brain imaging shows that my perfusion is much better—and it was good before. My test results for physiological, cognitive, and fitness are all much better and, again, I was pretty good sixteen years ago.

Just as we advise our clients, I make it a priority to exercise regularly, pushing hard for those hormesis benefits, and maintain a disciplined, healthy diet. Here is a quick summary of my fitness conditioning and diet regimen.

EXERCISE. I run a 10k (10 kilometers, or 6.2 miles) at an average pace under eight minutes per mile, or forty-five minutes total, three or four times a week. I ran my fastest time ever for a single run when I was age fifty-two, at thirty-nine minutes (average pace: six minutes, thirty seconds per mile). But it isn't good to always run your fastest, or go farther than a 10k, because eventually you will have trouble with your mechanics.

I train with hand weights and barbells to maintain or build upper-body mass. Mostly I do aerobic exercise to preserve and enhance cardiovascular–lung fitness—that is, bolster my heart, blood circulation, and lungs.

FASTING/NUTRITION. I follow a routine of not eating anything for sixteen hours, with an eight-hour window for eating—usually from late morning to early evening. I limit carbohydrates as much as possible—not eating bread, potatoes, white rice, or pasta often. I don't drink sugary sodas or other sweet beverages. I like good cheesecake and enjoy a slice occasionally.

I eat a lot of fresh vegetables and forest fruits such as raspberries, strawberries, and blueberries almost every meal. And a good Mediterranean salad with olive oil. I drink a lot of water, both tap and sparkling. I also drink four to five cups of coffee a day during the week, starting in the morning. This is my kind of sin, but I enjoy coffee.

On that note of self-indulgence, I am pleased to share the findings of an in vitro study. Contrary to assertions of people who claim coffee drinking is not healthy, certain compounds in espresso can inhibit the accumulation of tau protein. That's a wonderful thing. As we saw in chapter 10, tau protein is closely linked to the development of Alzheimer's disease.[1] On the weekend, for me, it's one or two cups, and that's it.

LOCATION. I go to the gym very early in the morning during the week. On weekends I like to jog outside at the beach or other places, which is a nice option when you live in Israel.

SLEEP. My goal is six hours each night, but I don't achieve that every night during the week because I am quite busy. It's more like five to six hours per night. During the day, I don't have time for naps. On Friday nights, I am tired and can sleep eight hours with a good, spontaneous wake-up in the morning. Saturday is usually closer to six hours.

MEDITATION. I can meditate only when I am in the chamber, not anywhere else. As I begin to focus on my breathing with the mask on, I start to see waves of lights coming; they go from the back to the front. It's an unbelievable experience. I love it. I meditate almost the entire two hours.

MENTAL OUTLOOK. I always try to focus my thoughts on the future, to look forward. When there is disagreement about something that already happened, I don't want to get into whose fault it is. All I want to know is what insights were gained and how we will apply those insights from here.

WE ALL MAKE MISTAKES. That's part of doing. Wise people try to make only new mistakes. As this blessing goes that I give to my young trainers and children, "I wish you will do as many mistakes as possible at the earliest stages of your career or life."

Conclusion

Today, the world of medical care is undergoing a profound transformation. More people are taking an active role in understanding and managing their own health. While they still value the guidance of healthcare professionals, they have become more discerning, exploring alternative perspectives and treatment options. The era of unquestioning faith in a physician's word is fading, making way for a more informed and engaged approach to healthcare.

Yet, we continue to struggle with a huge problem. Even as the United States continues to spend more than twice per capita than other Western countries on healthcare, the U.S. crisis in declining life expectancy has become more acute. Life expectancy in the U.S. is the lowest of any wealthy nation. Moreover, as of 2021, U.S. life expectancy ranked no. 43 globally, according to the World Bank—a precipitous drop from the low teens in 1980.

Higher spending and poorer life expectancy makes no sense. As the tragic mortality wave from COVID-19 subsides, for now, drug overdose, diabetes, suicide (highly correlated with PTSD), heart disease, and homicide remain brutal factors driving this crisis.

Attempting to treat disease *after* disease arises is much more costly and much less effective than preventing disease. We can prevent disease at lower overall costs by fortifying the body's natural physiological and biological wonders. This is the goal of enhanced medicine. We should embrace *regeneration* instead of battling the effects of *degeneration.*

Small Investments for a Healthier Society

It is not necessary to invest more public funds to reverse this alarming decline in life expectancy. We should instead redirect a small portion of the trillions of dollars funding medical programs each year.

We should encourage elected officials and other policymakers to create direct financial incentives for people to exercise more, to eat healthier foods, to avoid self-destructive drugs. We should build more fitness centers within walking distance of local populations and, instead of charging people to use them, *pay them* to use these centers regularly. Or encourage them to walk or run in their neighborhoods.

We should invest public funds to eliminate food deserts in underserved neighborhoods and communities, to coach people to buy and consume nutritious foods. We should pay people, reward them for gains they make in basic measures such as body mass index (BMI) or their ability to use oxygen at higher levels during exercise (VO_2 Max)— gains that we know from mountains of accumulating statistics will reduce the onset of chronic diseases. We should encourage people to work or volunteer as late in life as they are able . . . to wake each day with a purpose that contributes to their communities and gives their life meaning.

Costs for public spending on these and other health-promoting behaviors and activities would be vastly smaller than the savings that we would see in the national medical insurance system we have today.

A healthier society has less need for medical insurance payments; fewer people by the age of fifty-five would be draining resources from society with huge medical expenses—expenses healthy people subsidize through Medicare taxes and a soaring federal debt. A healthier society has more people living longer and working longer, productively, and paying taxes.

Love and friendship, the most important things in life, are free. Simple, healthy diet habits, regular exercise, and purpose—the most important things for health and performance—are free.

In Western societies, where the resources are available, we can incorporate HBOT and the hyperoxic–hypoxic paradox to go further. We can remove bottlenecks in a person's biology and elevate their performance to the highest levels they can achieve from whatever those levels are at the outset.

If we take advantage of the foundations of enhanced medicine, we can preserve our youthful biology through the years. Our world is filled with more people who are doing this—people chronologically in their eighties and nineties, and beyond.

These people help younger generations improve their future by continuing to build and apply the knowledge they have accumulated in their ongoing work lives. In the years ahead, more people will pass the century mark and be doing the same thing: making vital contributions to society.

These are the people who will have had the discipline to keep their diets healthy, their fitness active, and their physiology and mental agility young, and they are early adaptors of emerging scientifically proven interventions such as HBOT.

But not the people with poor diets and low fitness levels and who lack purpose and access to the practices of enhanced medicine. These people will continue to accumulate comorbidities wrongly associated—in my view—with the so-called "normal aging": the chronic diseases of diabetes, heart disease, stroke, dementia, frailty, and more.

Another group, elite performers, is determined to improve their physical and mental performance. Elite performers have always been among us, perhaps 5 percent of the general population. They want to get better. They want to be the best at what they do. They take advantage of whatever new technologies or medical breakthroughs are available.

Do you want to be your best self?

In the years ahead, the gap between how well and how long elite performers live in contrast to others enmeshed in poor diets and fitness habits on the pathway toward chronic disease is going to accelerate. We can expect the magnitude of the elite performers' contributions to society and future generations to accelerate as well.

The person at age 120 will have 120 years of life experience. Henry Kissinger's advice on China was still sought by U.S. presidents and members of Congress prior to his death in 2023. The winning bid for a lunch with Warren Buffett, age ninety-two in 2022, was $19 million. (Proceeds went to charity.)

We make choices every day that determine, as much as we can control, how well and how long we will live. If you have a warning from your physician that you should not eat carbohydrates, what will you do with that information? If you have a recommendation to stop drinking sugary drinks and eating processed foods, to lose weight, and to exercise more, what will you do with that?

One day you might walk past a 150-year-old person who is still young, engaged in a lively conversation with a companion. Then, on a park bench a few yards away, you'll see an overweight, diabetic fifty-year-old person who is old, in constant pain, walks with difficulty, cannot think straight, and, I would wager, probably has no capacity for sexual relations.

We are at a turning point in human evolution, an inexorable march toward two subspecies. We will see more people living at these extremes. It is sad, terrifying even, to consider how difficult life is and will be for people at the lower extreme. By age fifty, afflicted with various combinations of obesity, diabetes, stroke, and faltering cognitive ability, heart disease, and perhaps cancers, they will have begun the collapsing finale of their lifetimes.

And yet, most people are in the middle, certainly hundreds of millions of people. You or people you know may be among them. They represent a huge potential for humankind in the coming decades. These are people we can presume want to live healthier lives as they age. For myriad reasons they may be either uncertain or unmotivated about what to do.

These are the people that we in the medical professions and those of us already pursuing elite performance especially need to educate, push, and inspire. One hundred twenty years has been considered by most physicians and medical scientists to be the upper limit for human life. With the evolving science of enhanced medicine, we could probably reach for more.

Pushing the Boundaries of Enhanced Medicine

Many scientists, bolstered in recent years by a tsunami of private funding, continue to make intriguing discoveries that may extend the potential of human lifespan significantly. The scientific foundation of enhanced medicine continues to expand, with thousands of clients and patients experiencing revitalized biological performance. Our clinics, including the Sagol Center in Israel, along with the Aviv Clinics in central Florida and Dubai, have garnered growing interest.

You've heard inspiring stories of five men—Alon Day and Avishai Abrahami (Israel), Dr. Joseph Maroon (United States), and Dylan Hartley (United Kingdom) in chapter 2 and Patrick (Dubai) in chapter 9—who generously offered to share their experiences with enhanced medicine.

You've met some remarkable pioneers in our field—esteemed colleagues such as Amir Hadanny, Karen Doenyas-Barak, Rachel Lev-Wiesel, Shir Daphna-Tekoah, and Karin Elman-Shina. Together, with our research teams, we've published more than a hundred scientific papers. Each unravels a mystery of the hyperoxic–hypoxic paradox and the remarkable capacity of the human body to repair and regenerate.

Continuing research breakthroughs and a burgeoning trove of clinical data from clients and patients have established what we call the baseline of enhanced medicine. We have proved that enhanced medicine is not only possible but transformative.

A rising generation of researchers and physicians, a second wave, is devoting their careers now to further this science and its applications. These young medical scientists and physicians regard our research achievements as their starting point. Their fresh perspectives and unwavering dedication will push the boundaries of what we can achieve in treating brain injuries and elevating human performance.

Young minds are the greatest resource that we, *homo sapiens*, have on this planet. In time, we can expect more policymakers and healthcare professionals to join this rising tide.

Road Map for Better Health, Performance

As you think about what these realities and possibilities for rejuvenating human biology might mean for you personally, for your work, for your family and friends, let's revisit the same question we asked in chapter 11. If you could choose which age you would rather be, eighteen or seventy, which would you choose?

The focus for me in my research is biological performance, not necessarily extending longevity. When we understand the intricate complexities of nature—in this case, our human biology—we can measure and redirect it. We want to sustain healthy mental and physical capabilities all along our journey as we age. Living life worth living!

The rapid advances in enhanced medicine have opened new horizons for us all. It is my hope that this book has provided you with a clear and rigorous scientific road map to elevate your health and performance, a deeper understanding and appreciation of these transformative possibilities.

As we embrace the future of healthcare, remember that your journey to optimal health and performance starts today, from wherever you are, toward the highest potential attainable with the remarkable capabilities of your body and mind.

Acknowledgments

Among the many people who have played pivotal roles in my life and journey in medicine, I owe immense gratitude to my parents, immediate family, and the countless colleagues in science and medicine I've had the privilege of working alongside now for more than twenty years.

I could fill another book with stories to properly evoke and honor the many other guardians of my good fortune and stewards of new opportunities that shaped my path. But, before bowing out, let me mention three truly inspiring people who provided the most profound influence and unwavering support throughout my professional career: Professor Ahuva Golic, MD, industrialist Sami Sagol, and the late Professor Eshel Ben-Jacob.

PROFESSOR AHUVA GOLIC, MD: A distinguished clinician, Dr. Golic was medical director of internal medicine in the hospital where I served my residency. Known fondly as "Ahuva," her ability to connect with and genuinely care for her patients is unparalleled. I learned from Ahuva that there is no substitute for the human touch in medicine.

Listening attentively and having that physician's touch can often lead to a diagnosis in over 90 percent of cases, with sophisticated technologies and medical tests needed only for confirmation. These fundamental skills cannot be acquired solely through reading. Just as a carpenter's apprentice requires guidance from a master to craft a stable table or chair, a medical resident must work closely with their professor to acquire essential clinical skills. I am privileged to pass along the knowledge and practical insights I gained from Professor Ahuva—hopefully in a manner that honors her legacy—to the residents and medical colleagues under my mentorship.

SAMI SAGOL: A self-made industrialist who believed in my potential when I was developing my early research, Sami Sagol provided invaluable resources and insight that encouraged me to dream big. Born in Turkey, Sami immigrated to Israel at the age of fifteen. After his military service in the 1980s, he assumed leadership of Keter Plastics, his father Joseph's business, founded in 1948. Under Sami's guidance, the company evolved from a small local enterprise into a global industry leader in consumer products, employing 4,500 people worldwide.

Sami is the visionary behind Tel-Aviv University's Sagol School of Neuroscience, a pioneering interdisciplinary institution that unites brain studies across seven faculties at the university. With a vision to position Israel as a prominent international neuroscience hub, he established the Sagol International Network, comprising distinguished researchers from multiple universities and research institutes who collaborate in the field of neuroscience.

I can never express sufficient gratitude for Sami's first visit to my humble clinic-chamber. He had heard about a young physician who might be engaged in something intriguing, and he reached out to me. We engaged in thought-provoking discussions, and a few weeks later, he inquired, "Shai, what do you need?" and then he provided.

Sami's support extends beyond just resources; he imparted to me the inspiration to dream big, to forge ahead, to embrace mistakes, and to view failures as invisible stepping stones to success. Whenever I meet with Sami, regardless of how grand my dreams may be, he continues to challenge me to dream even bigger.

PROFESSOR ESHEL BEN-JACOB: A distinguished theoretical and experimental physicist at Tel Aviv University, professor Ben-Jacob held the Maguy-Glass Chair in Physics of Complex Systems, and at Rice University in Houston was a Fellow of the Center for Theoretical Biological Physics. I first met Eshel when Sami asked him to assess the scientific merit of my ideas and theories.

A few days after our first meeting, as I wrote in chapter 5, Eshel asked if he could spend a couple of days observing my work, explaining that he wanted to be my shadow during that time. Those "couple of days" evolved into years of collaborative work and a deep friendship. A trailblazer in the study of bacterial intelligence and social behaviors of bacteria, Professor Eshel is the most brilliant scientist I've ever encountered. I've greatly missed his guidance and friendship since his death in 2015.

Under his mentorship, I learned how to conduct intricate analyses, how to think critically and articulate scientific concepts, and, most importantly, how to muster the courage to challenge established paradigms. I carry with me his enduring wisdom that:

- *"The pure gold is not afraid of the melting mud."* When you possess clean source data, do not fear the criticism of conservative physicians, scientists, or regulators.

- *"Don't believe, challenge."* Do not merely accept what you were taught or what you have read; challenge it. The greatest impediment to progress in science and medicine lies in blind adherence to conventional teachings from school and university.

I also express my deepest gratitude to Noa Sobol, Michael Lobel, and Jonathan Preminger from AVIV Scientific. Their unwavering encouragement and support compelled me to embark on this journey of writing a book. Had I known how much time and effort it would demand from me at the outset, I might have hesitated. Yet, now that the project is complete, I find immense satisfaction and pride in the final outcome.

I'd also like to thank our team at Amplify Publishing Group—Naren Aryal, CEO and publisher; Brandon Coward and Gillian Barth, production editors; Rebecca Andersen, copyeditor; and Caitlin Schultheis and Josh Taggert, designers—which was superb.

Finally, I wish to extend my heartfelt thanks to Tom Hayes, whose invaluable guidance was instrumental in shaping this book. While I've authored numerous scientific articles in the past, writing a book, particularly one intended for a broader audience beyond the scientific community, presented new challenges. The process of organizing complex ideas and scientific knowledge in a manner accessible to the intelligent layperson is an art unto itself. Tom proved to be the ideal collaborator. He embodies the core principles of enhanced medicine in his practice.

My earnest hope is that our collective efforts have resulted in a work that effectively conveys the knowledge within these pages to our readers. Your pursuit of improved performance, applying the knowledge of enhanced medicine, is a noble endeavor. I am sincerely grateful for the opportunity to contribute to it.

About the Author

SHAI EFRATI, MD, is a renowned physician specializing in internal medicine, nephrology, and hyperbaric medicine. As the director of the Sagol Center for Hyperbaric Medicine and Research and the head of the nephrology unit at Shamir Medical Center, he leads the world's largest hyperbaric medicine center, which treats more than 350 patients each day.

Globally recognized for his expertise, he is also the author or co-author of more than 170 scientific publications and a sought-after speaker at international medical conferences. His pioneering research in neuroplasticity harnesses novel hyperbaric oxygen therapy protocols to promote brain and tissue repair, enhance cognitive function, and improve physical performance across all age groups.

Dr. Efrati earned his medical degree from Ben Gurion University in 2000, completed his residency at the Shamir Medical Center, serves as a professor at Tel Aviv University's medical school, and actively trains physicians and medical professionals from several countries in hyperbaric and enhanced medicine. He is also the co-founder and chairman of the medical advisory board of Aviv Scientific. He lives in Israel.

Notes

Chapter 2: Peak Performance

1 "Alon Day," World of EuroNASCAR, June 22, 2022.
2 J.C. Maroon, "The effect of hyperbaric oxygen therapy on cognition, performance, proteomics, and telomere length— The difference between zero and one: A case report," *Frontiers in Neurology* 13, (July 2022).
3 Dr. Joseph Maroon, interview by book collaborator Thomas C. Hayes, July 28, 2023.
4 J.C. Maroon, "Hyperbaric Oxygen for Better Brain Health: My Personal Journey to Florida's Aviv Hyperbaric Clinic," JosephMaroon.com, January 18, 2022.
5 Op. cit. Maroon interview.
6 Maroon, "Hyperbaric Oxygen for Better Brain Health: My Personal Journey to Florida's Aviv Hyperbaric Clinic."
7 Ibid.

8   Maroon, "The effect of hyperbaric oxygen therapy on cognition, performance, proteomics, and telomere length—The difference between zero and one: A case report."

9   "Neurosurgeon Shares Positive Results from the Aviv Medical Program: Dr. Maroon's Story," Video interview, Aviv Clinics, 3:09, May 25, 2022.

10   A. Hadanny, Y. Hachmo, D. Rozali, et al., "Effects of Hyperbaric Oxygen Therapy on Mitochondrial Respiration and Physical Performance in Middle-Aged Athletes: A Blinded, Randomized Controlled Trial," *Sports Medicine* 8, no. 22, (February 2022).

11   Avishai Abrahami, "Four Lessons I Wish I Learned Before Going Public," *Entrepreneur*, January 13, 2014.

Chapter 3. Fooling Our Bodies into Improving Themselves

1   Johns Hopkins Medicine, "Johns Hopkins Nobel Prize Award Winners," October 7, 2019.

2   Gina Kolata and Megan Specia, "Nobel Prize in Medicine Awarded for Research on How Cells Manage Oxygen," *New York Times*, October 7, 2019.

3   The Nobel Prize, "The Nobel Prize in Physiology or Medicine 2019," press release, October 7, 2019.

4   B. Gonzales-Portillo, T. Lippert, H. Ngyuen, J-Y Lee, and C. Borlongan, "Hyperbaric oxygen therapy: A new look on treating stroke and traumatic brain injury," *Brain Circulation* 5, no. 3, (September 2019): 101–105.

Chapter 4: The Brain as a Tissue

1   D. Vadas, L. Kalichmann, A. Hadanny, and S. Efrati, "Hyperbaric Oxygen Therapy Can Enhance Brain Activity and Multitasking Performance," *Frontiers in Integrative Neuroscience* 11, (September 2017).

2   Ibid.

3   Lulu Xie et al., "Sleep Drives Metabolic Clearance from the Adult Brain," *Science* 342, no. 6156, (October 2013).

Chapter 5: Stroke

1   The company is Hospitech Respiration Ltd. Founded in 2006, the medical device company specializes in airway management for patients in intensive care units (ICUs) and other hospital wards.

2   S. Efrati, G. Fishlev, Y. Bechor, O. Volkov, J. Bergan, K. Kliakhandler, I. Kamiager, N. Gal, M. Friedman, E. Ben-Jacob, and H. Golan, "Hyperbaric oxygen induces late neuroplasticity in post-stroke patients—randomized, prospective trial," *PLOS One* 8, no. 1, (January 2013).

3   The Centers for Disease Control and Prevention publish online a compilation of extensive data and medical advice regarding strokes and stroke prevention. "Stroke," Centers for Disease Control and Prevention, September 5, 2023.

4   Ibid.

5   S. Efrati, "Hyperbaric oxygen induces late neuroplasticity in post-stroke patients—randomized, prospective trial." The brain images in Figures 5-1 and 5-2 originally were published in this article about the clinical stroke study in 2013.

6   Ibid.

Chapter 6: Concussion

1   T.M. Andriessen, J. Horn, G. Franschman, J. van der Naalt, I. Haltsma, B. Jacobs, et al., "Epidemiology, severity classification, and outcome of moderate and severe traumatic brain injury: a prospective and multicenter study," *Journal of Neurotrauma* 28, no. 10, (2011): 2019–31.

2   D.M. Sosin, J.E. Sniezek, D.J. Thurman, "Incidence of mild and moderate brain injury in the United States, 1991," *Brain Injury* 10, no. 1, (1996): 47–54.

3   M. McDonagh, S. Carson, J. Ash, B.S. Russman, P.Z. Stavri, K.P. Krages, et al., "Hyperbaric oxygen therapy for brain injury, cerebral palsy, and stroke. Evidence report; technology assessment," *Medical Informatics and Clinical Epidemiology* 85, (2003):1–6.

4   University of Pittsburgh Medical Center, "Concussion Facts and Statistics."

5   The Sports Medicine Concussion Program at the University of Pittsburgh Medical Center evaluates more than 7,000 new cases of post-concussion syndrome (PCS) each year in person or virtually. A twenty-minute test for post-concussion analysis that Dr. Joseph Maroon created with a colleague—Are symptoms present? Are they severe?—is widely accepted as the standard for assessing sports-related concussions.

6   Studies conducted by the CTE Center at Boston University determined that the brains of several high-performing National Football League (NFL) players who took their own lives, such as Junior Seau, at age forty-three, Andre Waters, at forty-four, and Dave Duerson, at fifty, had evidence of CTE damage. More recently, the brain of Demaryius Thomas, a star receiver for the Denver Broncos who ended his life in 2021 at age thirty-three, was diagnosed with the disease. (CTE damage investigations are possible only after a person's death.) A 2017 analysis by the center determined that 110 of 111 brains of former NFL players showed signs of CTE. The high correlation likely stemmed from the fact that the brains of former players were donated by families who said the players had experienced episodes of symptoms associated with CTE.

7   Rahav Boussi-Gross et al., "Hyperbaric Oxygen Therapy Can Improve Post Concussion Syndrome Years after Mild Traumatic Brain Injury—Randomized Prospective Trial," *PLOS One*. 8, no. 11, (November 2013).

8   Paul G. Harch, Susan R. Andrews, Cara J. Rowe, Johannes R. Lischka, Mark H. Townsend, Qingzhao Yu, Donald E. Mercante, "Hyperbaric oxygen therapy for mild traumatic brain injury persistent postconcussion syndrome: a randomized controlled trial," *Medical Gas Research* 10, no. 1, (January–March 2020).

9   Eli Fried et al., "Persistent post-concussion syndrome in children after mild traumatic brain injury is prevalent and vastly underdiagnosed," *Scientific Reports* 12, no. 4364, (2022).

10 Andree-Ann Ledoux, PhD et al., "Risk of Mental Health Problems in Children and Youths Following Concussion," *JAMA Network Open* 5, no. 3, (March 2022).

11 Ibid.

Chapter 7: Fibromyalgia

1   Ilga Ruschak et al., "Fibromyalgia Syndrome Pain in Men and Women: A Scoping Review." *Healthcare (Basel)* 11, no. 2, (January 2023): 223.

2   M.B. Yunus, "The role of gender in fibromyalgia syndrome," *Current Rheumatology Reviews* 3, no. 2, (May 2001).

3   Arti Rana et al., "Traumatic Brain Injury Altered Normal Brain Signaling Pathways: Implications for Novel Therapeutics Approaches." *Current Neuropharmacology*, 17, no. 7, (June 2019): 614–629.

4   W Hauser MD, M-A. Fitzcharles MD, "Facts and myths pertaining to fibromyalgia," *Dialogues in Clinical Neuroscience,* 20, no. 1, (March 2018): 53–56.

5   Dan Buskila et al., "A painful train of events: Increased prevalence of fibromyalgia in survivors of a major train crash," *Clinical and Experimental Rheumatology* 27, 5 Suppl 56, (January 2009): S79–85.

6   Amir Hadanny et al., "Hyperbaric Oxygen Therapy Can Induce Neuroplasticity and Significant Clinical Improvement in Patients Suffering from Fibromyalgia with a History of Childhood Sexual Abuse—Randomized Controlled Trial," *Frontiers in Psychology* 9, (December 2018).

Chapter 8: Post-Traumatic Stress Disorder (PTSD)

1   Keren Doenyas-Barak, MD et al., "Hyperbaric Oxygen Therapy for Veterans with Treatment-resistant PTSD: A Longitudinal Follow-Up Study," *Military Medicine* 26, (November 2022).

2   Michael J. Ostacher and Adam S. Cifu, "Management of Posttraumatic Stress Disorder," *JAMA* 321, no. 2, (January 2019): 200–201.

3   K.C. Koenen et al., "Posttraumatic stress disorder in the World Mental Health Surveys," *Psychology Medicine* 47, 13, (October 2017): 2260–74.

4   M. Steenkamp, B Litz, and C. Marmara, "First-line Psychotherapies for Military-Related PTSD," *JAMA* 232, no. 7, (January 2020): 656–657.

Chapter 9: Long COVID: Mysteries, Discoveries, and Cures

1   World Health Organization, "Post COVID-19 condition (Long COVID)," December 7, 2022.

2   S.J. Yong and S. Liu, "Proposed subtypes of post-COVID-19 syndrome (or long-COVID) and their respective potential therapies," *Reviews in Medical Virology* 32, no. 4, (July 2022).

3   Claire Pomeroy, "A Tsunami of Disability Is Coming as a Result of 'Long COVID': We need to plan for a future where millions of survivors are chronically ill," *Scientific American,* July 2021.

4   World Health Organization, "Post COVID-19 condition (Long COVID)."

5   Shani Zilberman-Itskovich et al., "Hyperbaric oxygen therapy improves neurocognitive functions and symptoms of post-COVID condition: randomized controlled trial," *Scientific Reports* 12, no. 11252, (July 2022).

6   A. Bhaiyat et al., "Hyperbaric oxygen treatment for long coronavirus disease-19: A case report," *Journal of Medical Case Reports* 16, no. 80, (February 2022).

7   G. Douad, S. Lee, F. Alfaro-Almagro, C. Arthofer, C. Wang, P. McCarthy, F. Lange, J.L. Anderson, L. Griffanti, E.J.N. Duff, 2022. "SARS-CoV-2 is associated with changes in brain structure in UK Biobank," *Nature* 604, (March 2022): 697–707.

8   M. Catalogna, E. Sasson, A. Hadanny, Y. Parag, S. Zilberman-Itskovich, and S. Efrati, "Effects of hyperbaric oxygen therapy on functional and structural connectivity in post-COVID-19 condition patients: A randomized, sham-controlled trial," *NeuroImage: Clinical* 36, no. 103218, (October 2022).

9   M. Leitman, S. Fuchs, V. Tyomkin, et al., "The effect of hyperbaric oxygen therapy on myocardial function in post-COVID-19 syndrome patients: a randomized controlled trial," *Scientific Reports* 13, no. 9473, (2023).

Chapter 10: Alzheimer's Disease

1   Alzheimer's Association, "2023 Alzheimer's Disease Facts and Figures: Special Report," 2023.

2   Winston Wong, PharmD, "Economic burden of Alzheimer's disease and managed care considerations," *American Journal of Managed Care*. 26, no. 8, (August 2020).

3   Jack C. de la Torre, "Cerebral Perfusion Enhancing Interventions: A New Strategy for the Prevention of Alzheimer Dementia," *Brain Pathology*. 26, no. 5, (September 2016): 618–31.

4   N.R. Sims and M.F. Anderson, "Mitochondrial contributions to tissue damage in stroke," *Neurochemistry International* 40, no. 6, (May 2002): 511–526.

5   J.L. Yang, S. Mukda, and S.D. Chen, "Diverse roles of mitochondria in ischemic stroke," *Redox Biology* 16, (June 2018): 263–275.

6   Alzheimer's Association, "2023 Alzheimer's Disease Facts and Figures: Special Report," and Wong, "Economic burden of Alzheimer's disease and managed care considerations."

7   R. Pluta, S. Januszewski, S.J. Czuczwar, "Brain Ischemia as a Prelude to Alzheimer's Disease," *Front. Aging Neurosci,* 13, (February 2021): 636–653.

8   In January 2023, the U.S. Food and Drug Administration approved a drug that in mid-stage clinical trials slowed progression of Alzheimer's during mild cognitive impairment, the early stage of the illness. The drug, lecanemab, is a monoclonal antibody developed by two companies, Japan's Eisai and Biogen in the United States. It is being marketed as Leqembi.

9   K. Elman-Shina and S. Efrati, "Ischemia is a common trigger for Alzheimer's Disease," *Front. Aging Neurosci.,* 14, no. 26, (September 2022).

10 T. Ngandu et al., "A 2-year multidomain intervention of diet, exercise, cognitive training, and vascular risk monitoring versus control to prevent cognitive decline in at-risk elderly people (FINGER): a randomised controlled trial," *Lancet* 385, no. 9984, (June 2015): 2255–63.

11 F.Z. Caprio and F.A Sorond, "Cerebrovascular Disease: Primary and Secondary Stroke Prevention," *Medical Clinics of North America* 103, no. 2, (March 2019): 295–308.

12 Ibid; M. Saito et al., "Reduced long-term care cost by social participation among older Japanese adults: a prospective follow-up study in JAGES," *BMJ Open* 9, no. 3, (March 2019),

13 Ibid. Saito et al.

14 M. Rusek et al., "Ketogenic Diet in Alzheimer's Disease," *International Journal of Molecular Sciences* 20, no. 16, (August 2019); T. Ballarini et al., "Mediterranean Diet, Alzheimer Disease Biomarkers, and Brain Atrophy in Old Age," *Neurology* 96, no. 24, (May 2021).

15 C. Judge et al., "Aspiring for primary prevention of stroke in individuals without cardiovascular disease—A meta-analysis," *International Journal of Stroke* 15, no. 1, (June 2019).

16 M. Piegza et al., "Cognitive Functions in Patients after Carotid Artery Revascularization—A Narrative Review," *Brain Sciences* 11, no. 10, (October 2021).

17 M. Piegza et al., "Cognitive functions and sense of coherence in patients with carotid artery stenosis – Preliminary report," *Frontiers in Psychiatry*, 14 (September 2023); M. Kohta MD, PhD et, al.," Effects of carotid revascularization on cognitive function and brain functional connectivity in carotid stenosis patients with cognitive impairment: a pilot study," *Journal of Neurosurgery*, 139, no. 4, (March 2023): 1010–1017.

18 N. Kandia, P.A. Ong, et al., "Treatment of dementia and mild cognitive impairment with or without cerebrovascular disease: Expert consensus on the use of Ginkgo biloba extract, EGb 761®," *CNS Neuroscience and Therapeutics* 25, no. 2, (January 2019): 288–298.

19 W. Gulisano et al., "Role of Amyloid-beta and Tau Proteins in Alzheimer's Disease: Confuting the Amyloid Cascade," *Journal of Alzheimer's Disease* 68, no. 1, (March 2019): 415; S. Walsh et al., "Aducanumab for Alzheimer's Disease?" *BMJ* 374, no. 1682, (July 2021).

20 Erin E. Congdon and Einar M. Sigurdsson, "Tau-targeting therapies for Alzheimer disease," *Nature Reviews Neurology* 14, no. 7, (June 2018): 399–415.

21 Ibid.

22 Asher Mullard, "Anti-tau antibody failures stack up," *Nature Reviews Drug Discovery*, November 2, 2021.

23 R. Pluta et al., "Neuroprotective and Neurological/Cognitive Enhancement Effects of Curcumin after Brain Ischemia Injury with Alzheimer's Disease Phenotype," *International Journal of Molecular Sciences* 19, no. 12, (December 2018).

Chapter 11: Aging Is a Good Thing

1   Matt Lauer, "'Friends' Creators Share Show's Beginnings," NBC News, May 6, 2004.

2   National Center for Health Statistics, Centers for Disease Control and Prevention, "Life Expectancy in the U.S. Dropped for the Second Year in a Row in 2021," press release, August 31, 2022.

3   Laura Niedernhofer was one of four scientists featured in the World Science Festival video: "Life Expanded: The Scientific Quest for a Fountain of Youth," video, Word Science Festival, 1:26, April 28, 2022.

4   Elizabeth Blackburn and Elissa Epel, *The Telomere Effect: A Revolutionary Approach for Living Younger, Healthier, Longer* (Grand Central Publishing: New York, 2017).

5   Ibid.

6   Daniel J. Levitin, *Successful Aging: A Neuroscientist Explores the Power and Potential of Our Lives* (Dutton: New York, 2020): 313.

7   Justin Sonnenburg and Erica Sonnenburg, *The Good Gut: Taking Control of Your Weight, Your Mood, and Your Long-Term Health* (Penguin Press: New York, 2015).

Chapter 12: Retirement Is a Bad Thing

1   Friedrich Nietsche, *Twilight of the Idols, or, How to Philosophize with a Hammer* (Hackett Publishing Company: Indianapolis, IN, 1997).

Chapter 13: My Personal Regimen: HBOT, Fitness, Nutrition, and Diet

1   Roberto Tira et. al, "Espresso Coffee Mitigates the Aggregation and Condensation of Alzheimer's Associated Tau Protein" *Journal of Agricultural and Food Chemistry* 71, no. 30. (July 2023): 11429–11441.

Index

transcranial magnetic stimulation
(TMS), 89
traumatic brain injury (TBI), 45,
49-51, 89, 112–14, 115n, 116,
122, 124, 127, 150, 191
two atmospheres absolute (2 ATA),
58, 59

U
unhealthy diets, 217–19
University of Pittsburgh Medical
Center (UPMC), 30
UPMC. *See* University of Pittsburgh
Medical Center
U.S. Food & Drug Administration
(FDA), 147, 226

V
vaccination, 8–9, 12, 168
Vadas, Dor, 86
vascular endothelial growth factor
(VEG-F), 61, 64, 67, 72–73, 76,
77
vascular pathology, 184, 185
VEG-F. *See* vascular endothelial
growth factor
Veterans Affairs Department, 157
Veterans Health Administration, 157
VHLp. *See* von Hippel–Lindau
protein
visual motor cortex, 34
VO$_2$ Max (maximal oxygen efficiency
volume), 236
Alon's case, 24, 24n
Avishai's case, *42*
Dylan's case, 48
Patrick's case, 173
von Bismarck, Otto, 226

von Hippel–Lindau protein (VHLp),
66

W
weightiness, 146
whales, longevity of bowhead,
214–16
white matter lesions, 184, 191
WHO. *See* World Health
Organization
Wix.com, 39–40
World Health Organization (WHO),
167

X
Xie, Lulu, 88

Y
Yang, J. L., 183